WHY
PREGNANCY
AND POSTNATAL
EXERCISE
MATTER
Rehana Jawadwala

pinter
&
martin

Why Pregnancy and Postnatal Exercise Matter (Pinter & Martin Why It Matters 19)

First published by Pinter & Martin Ltd 2020

©2020 Rehana Jawadwala

ISBN 978-1-78066-620-4

Also available as an ebook

Pinter & Martin Why It Matters ISSN 2056-8657
Series editor: Susan Last
Index: Helen Bilton
Cover Design: Blok Graphic, London
Cover Illustration: Lucy Davey
Illustrations: Rees Wharton

British Library Cataloguing-in-Publication Data
A catalogue record for this book is available from the British Library.

Set in Minion

Printed and bound in the EU by Hussar

This book has been printed on paper that is sourced and harvested from sustainable forests and is FSC accredited.

Pinter & Martin Ltd
6 Effra Parade
London SW2 1PS

pinterandmartin.com

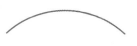

Contents

Disclaimer

Please note that this book provides general information about exercise and diet in pregnancy and the postnatal period, and does not constitute medical advice for individuals. Please consult your own healthcare providers when making decisions that may affect your health or that of your baby: the evidence and information discussed in this book may help you to have these conversations.

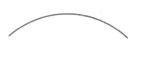

Author's Note

Before I had children, I was a girl who was so focused on helping athletes achieve medals that I never saw a buggy or a pregnant belly even if I ran into one on a busy high street: they just weren't on my radar. Until, of course, I became pregnant myself. Very quickly I came across physical and physiological roadblocks to my training – some of them, unbeknown to me, even before I took that pregnancy test. Then came the emotional and mental blocks: should I keep doing the physical training I was used to? Should I stop? Should I slow down? How much exercise is safe? What kind? Opinions ranged from 'rest it out in the first trimester due to the risk of miscarriage' to 'the universe will take care of your baby and you should carry on regardless'. Most of the advice seemed unfounded, biased and not evidence based. Thus I began to apply my scientific training to this deeply personal issue: maintaining my identity (through my physical activity) and caring for the baby growing inside me.

I read widely. I trained as a perinatal yoga teacher, and I engaged with anything that could inform me about how I could manage physical activity throughout my pregnancy and beyond. I was anxious about it until late pregnancy when my mind calmed and I was more convinced than ever that staying active was a good decision. I was not suffering from some of the common ailments pregnant women around me seemed to be enduring.

Then came the birth of my first daughter. Nothing had prepared me for the sheer physicality of birth. If someone like me, who prided herself on her physical strength, felt overwhelmed by it, what must more sedentary women, with a more relaxed approach to physical activity, go through? Why did no one tell me, that despite running marathons nothing would come close to the physical effort of birthing a baby, or the mental resilience required to adapt to motherhood?!

This was when my personal interest in perinatal exercise became a raging passion. As I dug into the topic, I realised the multiple and complex barriers there were to getting women to move more during pregnancy. I heard stories of scared women, and equally unfortunate stories of care providers who were unsure of the specifics of the advice they were meant to give, thus missing some great opportunities for intervention. That's when I knew I had to bring all my exercise physiology understanding to this topic and concentrate my energies on arguing for the profound impact of our lifestyle choices at this important time in our lives.

This book aims to present you with an overview of the evidence that illustrates the importance of physical activity throughout the perinatal period of a woman's life, when we feel so vulnerable, so responsible and so aware of the impact of each and every action. I hope this gives you the information you need to embark on an active pregnancy and transition to new motherhood with confidence.

I also hope this book convinces you that the impact of your choice to move more will have a long-term effect, not only on your own life and that of your baby, but for future generations. With the burden of lifestyle-related diseases ravaging our society, this small step (literally!) may change the path of our society in the years ahead. I hope you enjoy reading it.

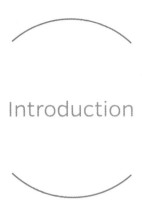

Introduction

Our life today is so different from only a few generations ago. Our lifestyle: our sedentary habit of driving long distances to sit at a desk for most of the day, eating our lunch without putting any effort into growing and making it, and our environment and culture which promotes productivity over relationships has very modern and shallow roots, unlike giving birth and rearing babies which has always been part of the human experience.

Is it a coincidence that we suffer during pregnancy with gestational diabetes and other such conditions? Is it a coincidence that we fear the physicality of birth? Is it a coincidence that we are seeing an exponential increase in metabolic diseases with each progressive generation?

As you will see, research indicates that none of these are coincidences. If we want to reverse this trend, which is adding hardships to our journey to becoming mothers, first and foremost we need to reframe how we think about pregnancy and motherhood, with its dated image of 'a vulnerable woman in a delicate condition'. We have spent hundreds of years perfecting this fallacy in a patriarchal culture. But you will see throughout this book that research has now revealed just how beneficial being active during our childbearing years can be.

This understanding has been slowly building, one small step at a time. Thus, despite the strength of the evidence, we are still only managing to say: 'It's okay to exercise during pregnancy', 'There are no adverse effects of exercise in pregnancy', and 'You can continue to exercise in pregnancy'. This is not enough for many women. Why, in 2020, are we tip-toeing around something so profoundly important for our own health and vitality and better outcomes for our children?

Saying it's okay to exercise during pregnancy and the postnatal period is not nearly enough, and women deserve better. We need to change the message and speak with a clear, assertive and empowering voice. It is *imperative* that we are encouraged to be physically active during our childbearing years.

In this book I explore what I consider to be three critical ideas:

1. How your physical activity will improve the quality of your life during pregnancy and the postnatal period.
2. Physical activity in the context of labour and birth outcomes.
3. The long-term health of our own and future generations.

When we are pregnant, we are often implored to do things for the sake of our growing baby; for example to eat better, or think about the medications we may be on. All of these decisions appeal to our altruistic mothering instincts. But if we embark on or continue with an active lifestyle during pregnancy, it has clear benefits for us as well as our babies, making pregnancy more comfortable and enjoyable. We do not need to submit to old wives' tales about pregnancy being an inevitable cause of back ache or urinary incontinence or sleepless nights. What if I told you that simply *spending less time sitting down* could reduce or even banish those banes of pregnancy? Or how powerful exercise can be in combatting stress, anxiety and depression, both during pregnancy and in the early days of new motherhood? Or that being active during pregnancy can make the process of birthing our babies safer, for them and for us? You might think I was pulling your leg, or overstating the case. But this is what the research is telling us.

Furthermore, and perhaps most important of all, simply by moving more we *affect the lives of our children*. This can be a gift like no other. The case for intergenerational health benefits from our lifestyle choices is now well-established, whereas only a decade or so ago it was just a theory. Whether you call it the 'developmental origins of health and disease', or 'early-life programming', it is about 'timing during the primal period' of our lives, as obstetrician Michel Odent has described it. If we are active during this crucial time, we convey health benefits to our babies by changing the way their genes will interact with the excesses of food, environmental pollutants and even stress that they will encounter throughout their entire lives. In some cases these benefits extend beyond one generation. This is both fascinating and hugely important for the health of mothers and babies.

Thus I invite you to examine the evidence, and feel confident in making small, meaningful changes to your life that will create a positive cycle of health for you and your family.

1

A brief history of pregnancy and postnatal exercise

Ladies who loll on sofas and easy chairs the greater part of the day and who seldom walk out have generally more lingering and severe labours than those females who attend to their household duties and take moderate and regular exercise in the open air.

This advice to pregnant women from the physician Pye Henry Chavasse in the 1800s was a break from the then current norm of treating pregnant women with anxious caution.[1] Chavasse was a proponent of breastfeeding and co-sleeping, cuddles and clothes that didn't corset women: he was a true original thinker and pioneer. He didn't have the scientific evidence that shows how keeping active throughout pregnancy can make the whole journey more enjoyable and labour less intense, nor did he know of the epigenetic advantages we can pass on to our children. Nevertheless, his observations led him to understand that being sedentary during pregnancy came with risks.

This anecdotal understanding is found in literature as far back as Aristotle. We see that a more active pregnancy, more ambulant labours, birthing stools and upright postures were the norm in childbirth advice.[2] It was not until the 1700s that the general ideology of the frailty of women (particularly privileged women) affected pregnancy and childbirth. These notions reinforced the prevalent gender roles and bias. At the time there was very little empirical evidence of the impact of pregnancy-related exercise on mother and baby. So it was a lot simpler to 'err on the side of caution' than to risk a pregnancy. Activities such as tennis, riding, swimming and cycling were all considered too violent for pregnant women in the 19th and 20th century.[3] The only things deemed 'safe' were gentle housework and a small amount of walking. However, reports dotted throughout the literature describe working-class and poor women as having easier births, thanks to their active lifestyle.

Interestingly, the idea of the frailty of women, and their pregnancies, was not questioned until the 1960s and the second wave of feminism, when we started to ask what was so violent about tennis?[4] And in the 1970s, with the health and fitness boom and an increased sense of freedom, came new studies that showed that exercise during pregnancy was safe. So the idea of the 'delicate pregnant woman' persisted for a long time in our culture, and we are still trying to break free from these constraints.

By the late 1970s and early 1980s, the move towards physical fitness for women was gaining pace. Our desire for ownership of our health, Jane Fonda's fabulous leg warmers and women becoming a niche market led academic researchers to sit up and take notice. Women wanted to be active during pregnancy, but we wanted to know if it was safe. In many ways we are still searching for answers.

Early studies were fraught with methodological short-comings and there were big gaps in basic understanding due to ethical and technological barriers. From these early investigations there arose some rudimentary unqualified theories about a lack of nutrients and oxygen for the foetus if the mother exercised. The increased requirements for blood supply to the muscles for exercise led people to hypothesise that this would rob the foetus of critical blood supply. Fears around miscarriage, premature rupture of membranes (waters), over-heating and foetal growth retardation were all theoretical constructs that had not been tested.

Slowly, research provided us with an understanding of how the body manages to adapt beautifully to the needs of both mother and baby. We began to get some good quality insights into the way that nature protects what it deems valuable. By the 1990s there was tentative agreement among most academics that exercise at moderate levels was safe during pregnancy, and simplistic guidelines began to emerge from official quarters.[5] These guidelines still had many shortcomings, mostly due to a lack of good quality data. For example, if the general advice for women was to rest during the first trimester for fear of causing a miscarriage, that made it hard to study exercise in the first trimester of pregnancy. This 'chicken and egg' situation has been one of the hardest hurdles to overcome. It was not until we could do research at a molecular and genetic level that we started to understand the real causes of miscarriage and could start to exempt women from blame.

In the last decade we have made great strides in our physiological, epigenetic and biomechanical understanding of exercise during pregnancy. Most importantly, we now recognise that not only is it safe to exercise during pregnancy, but more importantly a sedentary lifestyle is *detrimental* to both mother and baby. It is this newfound confidence in the amazing benefits of keeping active that should drive us forward. Clinically meaningful reductions in the risks of developing gestational diabetes and hypertension, more energy and less fatigue, fewer complications at birth, faster recovery, improved bone density postnatally and reduced risks of metabolic diseases for babies when they grow up are just some of the reasons exercise should not only be 'allowed' during pregnancy, but actively encouraged.

Barriers to exercise

It's not just a lack of knowledge about the benefits of exercise that is keeping us from moving more during pregnancy and beyond. We encounter genuine, serious and structural barriers to getting more physical activity in our lives. An online survey of about 1,000 women showed that almost half of the respondents reported decreasing physical activity when they became pregnant, with 12% stopping altogether.[6]

My jogging came to almost an instant halt when I got pregnant. My breasts were so sore, and I was constantly breathing heavily, even with small activities. I tried other classes but I soon started to worry about miscarriage and other complications, so I decided to simply just stop till I felt better to take up a bit of walking again towards the end of my second trimester. But by this time, I had lost a lot of my fitness levels and it all felt too hard. Anon

Of course there will be genuine physical, emotional and medical reasons for some to reduce or stop exercise during pregnancy, but for most of us those reasons are based in an entrenched fear of harming our baby, social conditioning that pregnancy is a frail and delicate state, and most importantly a lack of clear and authoritative guidance from our care providers.

I conducted a small survey for a previous publication for AIMS[7] within my network of mothers on social media. The survey asked several questions about barriers women faced to getting and staying more active during pregnancy. Of 57 respondents, 63% felt that their work and home commitments meant they gave less priority to physical activity. Could it be that without guidance from our care providers clearly stating the benefits of moving more during pregnancy, we don't prioritise to make sure we include physical activity in our lives?

Of course, we can't simply shift the blame from mothers to midwives. The issue is structural. There are no specially trained professionals in exercise prescription for the pregnancy/postnatal period in our core care teams. Thus it is not fair to expect our care providers to give us meaningful information and motivation to change our thinking and behaviours. They need the confidence, the knowledge and above all the resources to be able to play an integral part in our collective shift towards a more active pregnancy.

The missing blocks

Although we have come a long way from viewing pregnancy as a delicate time, we still need more specific guidance about exercise from official bodies. In addition, we need further specific guidance for niche groups such as athletes, and at the other end of the spectrum, for sedentary women who want to start to get more movement into their days during pregnancy. We also need more specific guidance for each trimester, so that we can understand the shifting nature of risk, if any, from early to late pregnancy.

In 2019 some excellent guidance on physical exercise during pregnancy was published in other parts of the world. Canada's guidance, for example, says that 'Physical activity is now seen as a critical part of a healthy pregnancy.'[8] This is clearly a step in the right direction as we move away from language and vocabulary like 'no adverse effects' that we have seen in the past. The idea that 'exercise will not harm our babies' is not discouraging. But, with weight of current evidence behind us, we should move to phrases that are *encouraging* rather than simply *not discouraging*. Positive vocabulary will help reassure women who want to exercise but encounter negative scaremongering, and will give us the confidence to approach physical activity with a sense of enjoyment and ownership.

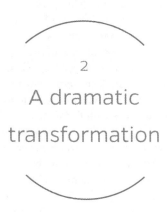

2

A dramatic transformation

There is no time in our lives more transformative than the period of pregnancy and birthing our babies. The transformation is dramatic both physically and mentally. But the outward manifestation of our changing bodies requires many new ways of coping with our pregnant selves. Simple acts like standing and sitting down can require adaptations.

Staying upright

Some postural changes during pregnancy are absolutely necessary to avoid toppling over. The way we achieve this is by moving our centre of gravity (COG). This is a hypothetical point on the body that holds the maximum concentration of our body weight upon which gravity can be most effective. COG changes at many points in our lives: when we get taller as kids, when we put on weight and when we get older and start to stoop.

In a non-pregnant person, standing COG is around the

navel. However, during pregnancy the expanding uterus displaces the COG, moving it forward, which could result in us falling forward in a front-heavy manner.

Essentially, the position of the uterus was in the perfect place, from a movement perspective, when our ancestors (chimps) were on all fours. The uterus, when expanded during pregnancy, simply hung lower to the ground and closer to gravity, causing no issues with the spine or moving about. As we slowly became upright, the uterus was no longer in the perfect place, as it extended outwards instead of closer to the ground to accommodate the growing baby.[1] To compensate for this, evolutionary adjustment modified the lower spine with a compensatory curve in, also known as lumbar lordosis. As pregnancy progresses this lordosis can become rather exaggerated, causing other anatomical changes (sometimes subtle) that impact not only movement and exercise, but may also cause pain and aches.

One of the most common ways to compensate for the

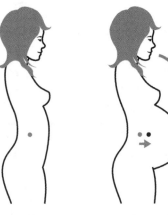

Normal spine   *No Lumbar Lordosis*

increased lumbar lordosis is by tilting the pelvis forward (anterior rotation) by approximately 5 degrees. This can create tension in the knees, shoulders and neck. Change in posture at the upper back, shoulders and neck can cause breathing restrictions that are mechanical, in addition to the physiological restrictions that already make breathing difficult during pregnancy. Thus, the spine and changing COG impact our ability to move and exercise.

Connecting the postural dots

To increase stability while moving, pregnant women do two things: we put more pressure on our heels (to compensate for the forward-moving COG) and we decrease our stride length.

Also, we tend to have both feet on the ground for longer. This allows for a more solid base of support (BOS). It also reduces the impact on the pelvis and the abdominal muscles. This leads to less range of movement (ROM) and over time decreases our capacity to move quickly, change position, turn and bend.

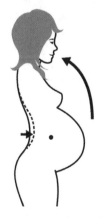

Pregnancy complete with Lumbar Lordosis

Thus, the basic postural changes that occur during pregnancy have three fundamental points of change: COG – BOS – ROM.

All three interact closely to impact our ability to function. Additionally, optimal posture and load transfer is important for the appropriate functioning of the joints and the load being placed on them. The transfer of correct load across the core (thorax cavity) is important to prevent the prolapse of internal organs and herniations. Our breathing is also greatly impacted by the way we distribute weight across our bodies, as suboptimal load transfer affects the movement of the ribcage, diaphragm range and pelvic stability while breathing.

Small differences

Most women who do not exercise do not notice these subtle postural changes as they are happening, and may only acknowledge them if pain or discomfort arise. However, reduced functional capacity of the musculoskeletal system also gives rise to conditions such as diastasis recti, generalised back pain, ligament strain, compression of the vertebral discs and so on.

> *I was very active before I got pregnant. Then everyone around me kept asking me to rest due to risk of miscarriage and I just stopped doing all my exercise. I felt very slow and tired too, but I think mostly I was scared of doing something wrong. I started again on my jogs when I was about 26 weeks and almost tripped the first time. This scared me and I stopped all the jogging till after my baby was born.* Frances

These changes also impact the fascia (connective tissue beneath the skin that stabilises, encloses, and separates muscles and other internal organs in our bodies). Myofascial changes due to improper postural alignment affect movement and muscular function not only during pregnancy, but also long after. Any changes to posture during pregnancy live on in the myofascial system, altering its stiffness and symmetry.

This affects the tension-support relationships in the bones and muscles, creating habits that may have long-term implications for the core, pelvic floor and breathing. A study looking at 7,800 women who had vaginal births showed that 31% of the women who had regained their continence in the early postnatal period (birth to one year) were incontinent 5–7 years later.[2] This study showed the long-term impact of bad posture and compensatory mechanisms that lead to long-term functional implications for women.

Muscular changes in pregnancy

Postural changes also make our muscles work a lot harder. If there is no awareness that the body is compensating, we tend to fall into certain habitual ways of moving that weaken some muscles and continue to strain others.

Thighs, hip flexors and deep muscles of the lower back all tend to tighten and shorten over the course of pregnancy. These muscles are heavily involved in standing, moving about and daily activities, and they are large muscles that need to stay strong and flexible to truly be able to take the impact of pregnancy weight changes.

Muscles of the buttocks, hamstrings (back of the thighs), the abdominal muscles, upper back and pelvic floor muscles, on the other hand, tend to weaken and over-stretch to compensate for tightness in the other areas of the body. Weakened abdominal muscles and the strain from the outward-growing uterus can cause the muscles to tear or strain, which is known as abdominus diastasis recti.

The above is a broad and general view of muscular changes in pregnancy: in fact these changes will be specific to each woman, based on your history of movement, anatomy and lifestyle.

Ligaments and joints in pregnancy

When your ligaments and joints relax as a response to hormonal changes during pregnancy (increasing amounts of oestrogen and relaxin), this puts pressure on your entire skeletomuscular system. These hormonal changes also affect water retention, and oedema (swelling) towards the end of the pregnancy can also affect movement.

The body can and does start to compensate for inefficient movement by placing the stress on other body parts. Postural and muscular changes increase the likelihood of joint injuries, for example in knees and ankles, in addition to back and spine pain.

Relaxation of the pelvic joints and ligaments is essential for your baby to pass through your birth canal. The effect of oestrogen, progesterone and relaxin on ligament and joint laxity starts as early as 6–8 weeks of pregnancy, and peaks at around 32–36 weeks of pregnancy.

A Cochrane review[2] in 2015 found that as many as 70–85% of pregnant women experience some pelvic or lower back pain associated with laxity. This is generally due to the stretching of the ligaments around the pelvis. When you bend or lift something off the ground your ligaments can cause inflammation in the pelvic area, leading to pain, which further reduces the stability of the pelvis and over time increases the possibility of asymmetrical ligament stretching causing further pelvic pain.

The ligaments around the uterus and abdomen also play a part in pain as the uterus stretches outwards. These big round and broad ligaments that surround and 'hold' the uterus if they are tight can make movement painful. Women who report pelvic girdle pain do not seem to have more or less laxity in their pelvis, but they do seem to have an asymmetrical laxity in the ligaments surrounding these joints.

Moving with grace

Exercise will allow you to understand, experience and embody your changing posture. When mild adjustments are needed, the body can easily adapt to these adjustments. When you continually keep active, you can experience the subtle changes in posture and alignment of your body during exercise, and your brain can make you aware of the adjustment needed. The role of a good exercise professional can be invaluable here, as they can externally observe and make suggestions about small changes to movement that will help you navigate your new body with more ease and confidence. If you have not stayed active, it will be harder for you to understand the nature of the adjustment your back, pelvis and spine can undergo, and eventually your posture will change according to your habitual ways of sitting or moving, which may not be conducive to a healthy alignment or movement.

> *I used to do a lot of ballet up until my university days when I gave up. I did go out and do a lot of dancing since. When I was pregnant with my first baby, I used to go to a specialist pregnancy Pilates class and realised that my core was not as strong as it used to be. My instructor was amazing. When we tried to do balances, she could spot who was compensating for their weak core and would straightaway correct us. Her subtle yet very observant style made me more graceful despite being pregnant and I almost felt like I was in ballet class again. I really enjoyed how easy it felt despite my growing bump.* Charlie-May

Risk of falling with changing COG in pregnancy

Very specific changes to the muscles and posture do increase the risk of falling while pregnant. The forces your muscles can produce reduce in efficiency due to the changes in posture and cause increased fatigue, which is one potential reason for the increased risk. While studying the gait of pregnant women during different trimesters, researchers found that pregnant women walk with a wider stance, use shorter strides and tend to push their tail bone out to compensate for the shift in COG. Exercise has been shown to reduce the risk of falling, as women who exercise have more range of movement in their torso, which makes it less rigid.[3] This ability to move the torso with greater flexibility and withstand greater strides reduces the risk of falling. Imagine the torso being flexible like a blade of grass rather than a rigid tree trunk: this ability to self-correct any postural anomalies during pregnancy is protective against falls.

Physiological changes
Changes in our breathing

Our breathing responds to our need for oxygen at any given point. When we need more oxygen our breathing changes to accommodate that need. This involves several aspects of our physiology that are all interconnected:

- Firstly, the physical space that we breathe in – lungs, thoracic cavity (rib cage and abdomen area), diaphragm movement and the general skeletal space around the ribcage. The amount of total oxygen we can get from the environment depends on the lungs' capacity to take in appropriate breaths.
- Secondly, how oxygen from the breath is transported across to the cells of the body via our blood circulation.
- And lastly, the role of certain hormones in influencing breathing and circulation, especially when these hormones change dramatically during pregnancy and the postnatal period.

When you get pregnant these three aspects interact to create an efficient maternal response to your and your baby's need for increased oxygen. Let's consider each one of them and the changes these systems go through during pregnancy to really understand the limitations we may face during physical activity while pregnant.

Preparing for higher oxygen needs

As early as 1–2 weeks after conception your body begins to adapt in preparation for the growth needs of your baby. Thus, many of us experience the effects of these changes before we are even aware that we might be pregnant. Some of the earliest adaptations come from the metabolic needs of the foetus in terms of oxygen and nutrients.

I remember the precise moment I thought I was pregnant. We were on holiday and my two-year-old son started to run off the pavement on to the street. I only ran a few steps to grab him back to safety, but I was completely out of breath. This happened to me the first time as well. I took a pregnancy test and it was positive. It's like being out of breath was the very first symptom I have had in both my pregnancies. Lorna

A study from 1988 studied 20 women in pre-pregnancy and then again at 7 and 15 weeks post-conception.[4] By the seventh week the researchers saw an 11% increase in plasma volume. This increase in blood volume is not accompanied by an increase in red blood cells at this point. This is the main reason why women very early in pregnancy may experience hyperventilation (an out-of-breath feeling). It is the early impact of progesterone and prostaglandins on the maternal system that makes us ventilate more than usual. During early pregnancy women tend to start taking bigger breaths without having to breathe faster to maintain oxygen intake. Research shows that this increase in ventilation can be as much as 24% of pre-pregnancy rates in early pregnancy and can reach more than 50% by late pregnancy.

Early pregnancy

Apart from ventilation, your heart rate gets faster too. This is because the red blood cells which carry oxygen do not increase proportionally with the increase in blood volume. The heart must distribute a greater volume of blood without a concurrent increase in oxygen supply. To compensate, the heart rate gets faster (to pump more blood around the body) and blood pressure reduces (to allow the arteries to carry this blood more freely). James Clapp, a pioneer in studies of exercise in pregnancy, found that heart rate increased by approximately 13 beats per minute (16%) at rest and blood pressure reduced by 8mmHg (9%) by the seventh week of pregnancy.[4]

So until red blood cell and haemoglobin levels increase, allowing for more oxygen to be transported, the body must compensate via hyperventilation, increased heart rate and decreased blood pressure in order to maintain oxygen needs. Because these changes occur before the foetus needs substantially higher amounts of oxygen, in the early days the maternal system is adjusting to a future need. Once the increased blood (plasma) volume matches an increase in red blood cells, breathing need not be so laboured. However, during this time, when the oxygen-carrying capacity of the cardiovascular system is under strain, you might find that any form of physical activity might become challenging.

Most women find these changes a big barrier to exercise. You may recognise them as feeling tired after only a little activity, or not being able to do exercises at the same intensity as before pregnancy. Remember that this feeling is a mechanism to protect the early neural and organ development of the foetus from excessive carbon dioxide (acidosis), which is produced as a by-product of exercise.

Late pregnancy

Towards the end of pregnancy the distention of the uterus becomes a physical barrier to breathing. Your diaphragm is pushed upwards, meaning the lungs cannot stretch downwards. However, the extra sideways expansion of the rib cage in pregnancy compensates, so your lung capacity can stay the same. If you experience some shortness of breath towards the end of your pregnancy there is nothing to worry about, and it should not stop you from engaging in physical pursuits that you enjoy.

Higher oxygen needs for increased oxygen consumption

It's not just breathing, but also the amount of blood that your system can circulate that affects the oxygen supply to your baby. Your cardiac output (the amount of blood the body pumps in one minute) increases dramatically in the first 16–20 weeks and then stays high (almost 40% higher) throughout pregnancy and into the early postpartum period.[5]

The increased blood is required to supply the placenta with nutrients and collect waste (approximately 80% of the increase in cardiac output goes to uterine blood flow). The rest is distributed to your kidneys for removal of waste metabolic products (which increase as a function of growing a baby) and to your skin to maintain core body temperature.

During exercise, cardiac output is maintained or even increased as the blood supplies nutrients and oxygen to additional muscles. A mother who exercised before pregnancy

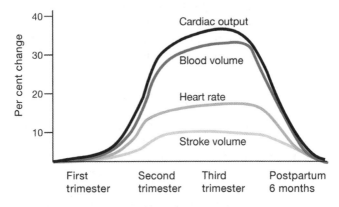

Cardiovascular changes during pregnancy and 6 months postpartum.

already has good compensatory mechanisms. Her placenta is better able to extract oxygen even when a small amount of blood is being redistributed from the uterus to her muscles. This is well maintained during exercise and then the full blood supply returns quickly to the uterus as exercise comes to an end. Thus, maintaining physical activity when you are trying to get pregnant has major rewards.

As your baby grows and the demand for oxygen continues to increase, the blood's oxygen-carrying capacity also starts to increase. Iron needs increase and more haemoglobin is formed. This haemoglobin is better at carrying oxygen in pregnancy than when not pregnant. Your baby's system also becomes better at oxygen extraction. All these adaptations mean that exercising does not cause any danger to the foetus during pregnancy in terms of being able to receive a healthy oxygen supply.

It is only when we exercise to an intensity that is so high that cardiac output is compromised and blood pH (acidosis) drops that the baby might experience distress due to maternal exercise. You would need to do an activity at more than 90% of your maximal capacity continuously for more than 20–30 minutes in order to attain such a state (which can probably only be achieved by well trained, professional athletes).[6] So normal physical activity, at moderate intensity for about 30–40 minutes, is not a danger to the baby throughout pregnancy, including the first trimester.

Hormones and fluid balance

As early as a couple of weeks after conception, the hormone HCG (human chorionic gonadotropin) and other related pregnancy hormones exert their influence on fluid balance and retention. Thirst increases during the early days of pregnancy, and women retain 6–8 litres more water than usual. Once relaxin starts to build up in the body from the end of the first trimester it promotes further water retention. Throughout pregnancy progesterone, oestrogen and relaxin all affect water balance. These hormones also play a role in pregnancy oedema (the accumulation of excessive watery fluids in tissues, leading to swelling).

We will talk about hydration later, but it is worth remembering that you will have an improved capacity to regulate your core body temperature, partly due to more dilated blood vessels and partly due to better sweating capacity. This is how your baby is shielded from the detrimental effects of increased core body temperature.

Changes to sleep in pregnancy

Lack of sleep impacts the quality your of life and the growth of your baby. Disturbed sleep is very common during pregnancy. More than 70–80% of pregnant women report disturbed sleep at some point in their pregnancy, with insufficient night sleep or significant daytime drowsiness.[7] We don't know if pregnancy and pregnancy hormones cause disturbed sleep, or whether other factors such as worry and stress play a bigger role. Insomnia, sleep-disordered breathing, restless leg syndrome, uncomfortable sleep positions and frequent urination all remain potent factors in disturbing sleep patterns during pregnancy.

Research suggests there is a U-shaped curve of sleep disturbances during pregnancy, with sleep latency (amount of time it takes to fall asleep after going to bed), efficiency (time in bed spent sleeping) and duration all getting a bit better for a short period during the second trimester. In the first trimester sleep disturbances are caused by hormones, whereas the disturbances in sleep towards the end of pregnancy are more about postural and bodily discomforts.

Your lack of sleep impacts the baby too. One study showed that women who slept for less than six hours a night for more than five days a week had a five times higher risk of c-section compared to women who had less than six hours a night for less than two days a week.[8] Another study has reported shorter labours in women who reported more than seven hours of sleep a night.[9]

Magic melatonin

Being physically active has a secret doorway into better sleep. A physically active lifestyle has shown to improve sleep quality, latency and efficiency.[10] This happens due to increased production of the hormone melatonin when we exercise. Melatonin is one of the primary modulators for sleep and influences circadian rhythms in both mother and foetus. It helps build clear day-night rhythms by syncing foetal heart rates with maternal activity-rest patterns, heart rate and body temperature along with maternal melatonin levels. Physical activity impacts all these parameters and helps amplify the co-ordination of foetal circadian rhythms.

Melatonin is also a potent antioxidant and the stress of physical activity helps increase melatonin activity. The antioxidant effects of melatonin have a possible protective impact on early miscarriages where increased free radical (oxidant) production can reduce the viability of the placenta. Thus, contrary to old beliefs, exercise may protect against miscarriages that occur due to placental viability. Maternal melatonin production also inhibits foetal cortisol production, allowing your growing baby to not only withstand the stress of your exercise, but also adjust his own future stress response to his external environment after birth.

I found sleeping well was almost impossible during pregnancy. I tried everything, no screens, baths and camomile tea. To be honest the only nights I really slept well were the evenings when I went to yoga. I think the exercise, relaxation at the end and the heavenly smells in the room all put me in a great place to go home and sleep well... sometimes I fell asleep on the mat towards the end. Shruti

Melatonin is also important in regulating blood pressure, which plays an important role in regulating oxygen and nutrient supply to your baby when you exercise. The blood pressure lowering effect of melatonin reduces the risk of pre-eclampsia and eclampsia.

Melatonin affects several physiological functions and is now considered an important player in the initiation and progress of labour. This is possibly one of the reasons why pregnant women who display poor sleep quality have more adverse birth-related outcomes. In 2004 Miller showed that mice which lacked melatonin regulation failed to get into established labour or were in unproductive labour for a long period.[11] We too have evolved to gauge labour timing and using our circadian rhythms, as it was safer to give birth in a den at night than in the fields during the day.

Thus, the various hormones that affect pregnancy and birth are impacted by physical activity. This co-ordinated regulation of all our physiological responses to maintaining pregnancy and facilitating birth shows that our bodies have extremely well-adapted ways of ensuring the health and viability of our pregnancies. Physical exercise facilitates this regulation. In the next chapter we'll look at the various forms of exercise available to us and how they relate to a healthier pregnancy, birth outcome and beneficial postnatal recovery.

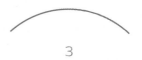

3

Ways to incorporate physical activity

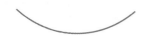

In the most simplistic way, aerobic training helps us lose stored body fat, resistance training helps us increase our muscle and flexibility, and mobility exercises help us navigate these two with poise. Combining a variety of exercises is the cornerstone of ensuring that we stay fit, gain appropriate amounts of weight during pregnancy and maintain a healthy body composition that will influence our metabolic hormones, such as insulin, to prevent complications such as gestational diabetes mellitus (GDM) and hypertension.

Postnatally these same principles of exercise will allow us to return to a lower body weight with a healthy body composition, while building fitness.

Aerobic and endurance exercise

It is now clear from good quality long-term studies that aerobic exercise during pregnancy does not cause any harm to mothers or babies. Evidence from recent literature in the field of epigenetics suggests that not only does aerobic exercise not cause any harm during pregnancy, but it is also absolutely essential for your and your baby's long-term health.[1]

Aerobic exercise is any exercise that needs oxygen to supply its energy demands. If we run, cycle or swim, for example, we need a continuous supply of oxygen to sustain these rhythmic activities over a long (more than a few minutes) period of time. Oxygen can only be supplied via blood, and thus the activity of the cardiovascular system becomes paramount in aerobic exercise. In addition, the fuel needed to sustain the activity mostly comes from blood glucose and fat (triglycerides). The slower the activity, the more fat we can use. Body fat is a complex molecule compared to carbohydrates and takes longer to break down, but it provides sustained energy. This is the principal reason why aerobic activity over a long period of time will help us reduce our body fat percentage.

If you have been running, jogging, cycling or doing other aerobic activities before you get pregnant, you will want to ensure that you can maintain some of that endurance and aerobic fitness through your pregnancy in order to be able to continue these activities after you have had your baby. In most cases this is achievable, and you should be encouraged. However, some physiological adaptations of pregnancy may impact your aerobic exercise capacity during pregnancy.

Changes in pregnancy that impact aerobic exercise

As we have seen, one of the first changes of pregnancy will be to your blood volume. There is a considerable increase in the water content of the blood, which reduces the number of red blood cells per litre of blood. This reduces the ability of your cardiovascular system to provide enough oxygen, manifesting in shortness of breath. So you may find that the intensity of run or swim you can manage decreases as a consequence.

Changes in breast tissue may mean that they are tender and become painful when running or jogging, especially without good support bras. The breasts may become fuller and uncomfortable and may take a few weeks or months to settle down.

Water retention and swelling can impact joints and cause an overall feeling of heaviness that may make you feel sluggish and slower in your activities.

> *I was so active before I was pregnant and found it very frustrating, and even felt a bit guilty, at not being able to continue running, biking etc. because I really wanted to keep active, I kept trying and after about 12 weeks I started going swimming a few times a week and that really helped.* Claire

The hormone relaxin peaks in the first 20 weeks of pregnancy and stays high throughout the remainder of the pregnancy. This may affect your joints and ligaments, compromising the stability of the exercise movements. The efficiency of your run or swim may decrease due to the micro-adjustments you will need to make to do the same movements as you did before becoming pregnant. For some women this can result in painful joints. So be aware of these small changes and consider complementing your aerobic exercise with strength training and flexibility and mobility work, to protect your capacity to exercise throughout your pregnancy, and also against long-term injury so you can return to your fitness levels post pregnancy.

High-impact aerobics

Running involves having both feet off the ground simultaneously, repeatedly over long periods. This increases the intensity of forces that travel up through the limbs into your pelvis. The soft tissues of the uterus and pelvic floor muscles can affect the integrity of your cervix. Recent research conducted with almost 1,300 women from 450 parks participating in parkrun has shown that regular running during pregnancy did not increase or decrease gestation period or onset of labour.[2] However, it significantly increased the chances of instrumental birth in women who ran throughout their pregnancy compared to women who stopped running during pregnancy. A possible explanation for this, although we don't have enough evidence at the moment, could be the impact of running on the cervix (the contrecoup effect – the cervix being impacted internally due to the forces generated through running) or the pelvic floor musculature being more rigid due to its role in core stability during high-impact activities such as running.

High-impact activities such as running also have an impact on urinary continence, even in non-pregnant women. It is important to consider the effect of pregnancy weight on the pelvic floor muscles and urinary and faecal continence. This becomes more of an issue for women who have had previous births.

Measuring the intensity of your aerobic exercise

How hard your heart needs to work for a particular exercise determines the intensity of the exercise for you. As each of our hearts will respond differently to the same exercise, we cannot expect our heart rates to be the same for the same activity. There are some sources on the internet which suggest keeping the heart rate below 140bpm during pregnancy. However, such absolute figures do not reflect each individual woman's capacity. An Olympic athlete might find running at 10 miles an hour a breeze and that might not tax her heart, but many of us would find that speed intensive. Thus, the evidence does not support keeping to a fixed heart rate. The guidance infographic published by the UK Department of Health does not state a single heart rate value, but simply mentions 'moderate intensity' exercise. This means you need to exercise at 'your' moderate intensity, which translates to mostly being able to speak in full sentences as you run or jog.

The 'talk test', as this is called, is a really a good indicator of exercise intensity and is easier than trying to measure your heart rate. Another variation of the talk test is the 'rate of perceived exertion scale', also known as 'Borg's intensity scale'. This is a scale from 6–20 and you rate how intense an exercise feels for you. At 6 you feel relaxed (as in sitting down relaxing), and at 20 you cannot do it anymore and must stop now. Once you get the hang of the scale you can give yourself a rating every now and then during exercise and adjust your speed according to the answer you get. The more you practice this technique, the more accurately the answers will tally with your heart rate capacity. In fact, this technique has stood the test of time so well that it is a well-known research tool.

Sometimes you will see a relative intensity stated, such as a percentage of maximal heart rate, or maximal exercise capacity. Generally during pregnancy staying below 90% of your maximal capacity has been shown to be a good idea, as there are reports of foetal distress over that capacity.[4] A range of 60–80% is sufficient to bring about the beneficial adaptations for your body and your health and birth outcomes (see Chapter 7), as well as the long-term health of your baby (see Chapter 8).

However, in order to understand what 60 or 80% of your maximal heart rate would be, the ideal way is to do a test of maximal intensity in a lab and then work out the percentage of the maximal heart rate you achieve. These tests are used in research as researchers can easily compare individual's results. However, the test of maximal capacity is not possible for most pregnant women! Another way is using a formula to work out your maximal heart rate, but that too has limitations.

The most common formula, with the fewest assumptions, takes into account your resting heart rate (which is a marker of your fitness level: the slower your resting heart rate, the more efficient your heart is). You can measure this after lying down for 15 minutes or before you get out of bed in the morning. Measure it anywhere you can find a strong pulse, such as your wrist or under your chin and slightly to one side (carotid artery pulse). You also need your assumed maximal heart rate, which is 220 minus your age (this formula assumes that the younger you are, the fitter you are – it does not take into account an older fitter person's heart rate, or a young and unfit person's).

Target Heart Rate =
[(max HR – resting HR) × %Intensity] + resting HR

If you don't want to calculate this yourself, you can search for 'Karvonen Heart Rate Calculator' on the internet. There are numerous sites that offer you a quick way to know what heart rate you need to stick to in order to exercise at 60–80% intensity or lower. The next issue you will have is making sure you take your pulse at regular intervals while you exercise.

If you find that calculations and measuring kill your passion for exercise, the best thing to do is use the talk test or practice the perceived intensity scale. These are both good measures of your exercise intensity and will give you the confidence to exercise within the healthy range for your body.

Strength and resistance-based exercise

Most research on strength and resistance training during pregnancy and the postnatal period indicates that these are safe forms of exercise. Resistance training – or weight training, as it is generally known – used to be considered unsafe during pregnancy. This is slowly changing thanks to good quality research data indicating otherwise. More and more women now engage in weight training or other high-intensity weight-bearing exercises before they get pregnant, and they want to know if it is safe to continue once they get pregnant.

Any training that challenges our muscular strength, using our own body weight or other kinds of weight resistance like bands, dumbbells or sandbags, is resistance training. This simply means that we use 'weights' – either our own body weight or external weights – to create stress on our muscles. By lifting this weight against gravity our body has to use the relevant muscles effectively to generate enough force to be able to do the task. This force is mostly generated by our 'fast twitch' or 'white' muscles. These are muscle fibres that generally cannot use oxygen as a source of energy. Thus, the effect of resistance training on physiological adaptations is rather different to aerobic exercise, which mostly uses the 'red' or 'slow twitch' muscles. Aer-obic (in the presence of oxygen) exercise uses oxygen to generate energy from food, and can use fuels such as carbohydrates and fats from the blood or from tissues such as fat stores in our body. But when we engage in resistance exercise, it is 'an-aerobic' (without oxygen) exercise. The fuel needed for muscular contraction is 'local' – such as the stored carbohydrates in the muscles (glycogen).

In order to mobilise local stores of muscle glycogen, the hormonal cascade is different to aerobic exercise. Resistance exercise in particular has been shown to be effective in reducing the risk of gestational diabetes,[5] because strength training induces adaptations in the muscles that mean they can utilise carbohydrates more efficiently. In addition, strength training also bypasses the insulin-based sugar clearance pathway by activating an enzyme called AMPK, making it an effective GDM management strategy.

Exercises that involve large muscle groups such as squats and lunges help in strengthening the core, maintaining functional strength and posture. It is important to remember when we do resistance exercise that blood pressure rises higher than normal for the duration of the exercise. We can mitigate this increase in blood pressure by incorporating appropriate rest periods during the exercise.

Repetitions and sets are also important considerations for a pregnant woman doing weights. Research indicates that moderate weight training has no adverse effects on the pregnancy or the foetus. Avoid lifting weights where you cannot do 15–20 repetitions. Only do 2–3 sets, and make sure you stay hydrated before, during and after exercise.

One important aspect of high-intensity weight training is the breathing pattern employed. Traditionally, in order to lift a heavy weight correctly, we would use the power of our core (trunk). This is even more effective if we can hold most of the core muscles and ligaments in a strong, connected way. A natural way to achieve this is to hold our breath for the duration of the lift, also known as the Valsalva manoeuvre. This can create an oxygen deficit in the body for a short period, which is tolerable in a non-pregnant state but probably not a good idea during pregnancy, as it can affect the oxygen supply to the foetus and cause distress. This is another reason not to train at more than 90% of your max capacity and to keep repetitions high instead of increasing the load (heavier weights). Smaller loads will allow you to breathe continuously throughout the repetitions.

Research indicates that resistance training performed one to three times a week helps improve muscular strength and increase lean mass, which helps maintain better body composition throughout pregnancy.[6] This level of frequency also ensures we allow time for our muscles and other tissues to recover from the exercise, so we are not loading our system with more stress. Every time you train your muscles to take a certain amount of load, by the end of the exercise the muscle fibres will have small amounts of 'micro tears' in them. This muscle breakdown initiates a cascade of growth and repair, which in turn increases muscle strength and adaptability.

I went to the gym a lot before I got pregnant. When I was still going to the gym in my second and third trimester, I got a lot of funny stares and some well-meaning people even accused me of not caring for my baby and being selfish and shallow for continuing my weight training. I had already modified my training and had slowed right down, but they didn't know that. I am not someone who can easily argue back so I kept quiet, but inside all these voices started to scare me. What if they were right? I thought I had done my research and nothing indicated that weight training was not okay during pregnancy. Also, all these women on social media were lifting really heavy weights. It was a confusing time to be honest. There was no clear guidance from any of the trainers in the gym either. They supported me but they never once said I was doing the right thing for my health and my baby. I wish people didn't accuse pregnant women of being selfish because they exercise in pregnancy, that is so wrong and so demoralising. Anon

Excessive (more than 15kg for a woman with normal BMI)

pregnancy weight gain has implications for maternal health, the birth and the infant. Pregnant women who engage in weight training avoid excessive fat storage and have a better body composition, which in turn helps maintain better insulin management and leads to a lower risk of developing gestational diabetes.[7] Resistance training also mitigates the risk of falling or injury as balance improves with better muscular function and strength.

How does your baby respond to resistance training?

A small but transient foetal heart rate increase is generally noticed when healthy, low-risk mothers exercise. A similar pattern is seen in resistance exercise, indicating that the foetus can tolerate both aerobic and resistance exercise in a similar way to healthy mothers. Some studies have indicated a transient 7–10 bpm increase in foetal heart rate after resistance exercise, which returns to normal within two minutes of the exercise ending.[8] However, there is a reverse trend observed in high-risk women, where bradycardia (lowering of the heart rate) is observed in response to resistance exercise.

However, it is important to reiterate that an isolated case of bradycardia in a low-risk pregnancy is not considered harmful for the baby. It is only consistent bradycardia after intense exercise that should be of concern. This generally occurs in women who have been sedentary or who do too much exercise (heavy lifting) without appropriate training adaptations.

Blood flow to the uterus may be compromised only if you lift very heavy weights (less than 10 repetitions per set, which leads to fatigue). This too is transient and in well-trained women there has been no reported long-term harm to the foetus.

Water-based exercise

Swimming and exercising in water is very popular with pregnant women in all stages of pregnancy. Water creates a certain buoyancy which can relieve pregnancy-related aches by making the pregnancy weight feel lighter for the duration of the immersion. Pregnant women report lower fatigue levels at the same intensity of exercise due to the buoyancy of water and their body temperature rising more slowly.

Research in the 1960s and 1970s increased our understanding of the effects of immersion in water during pregnancy. Scientists wanted to know if immersion in water increased blood volume, and whether as a consequence the pressure in the arteries would decrease. This thinking was driven by a desire to use water as a management strategy for pre-eclampsia. When you immerse yourself in water, almost immediately there is a redistribution of your fluids from the tissues into the blood. Plasma volume increases, causing a cascade of hormonal effects that increases diuresis (urine production). This is beneficial if you suffer from oedema, as the fluids retained in the extracellular space (swelling of ankles for example) are redistributed into the blood. Diuresis is more pronounced in standing postures, such as during aqua aerobics or jogging in the water, as the hydrostatic pressure in the lower limbs will increase the drainage of fluids from the ankles.

This increased urine output, combined with a potential increase in sweat production (which can go unnoticed), means that your fluid needs when you swim or exercise in water need particular attention. Body weight reduction of 0.5 to 0.8kg in pregnant women after two or more hours of water immersion has been noted in the literature.[9] This loss of body weight relates to loss of fluids. Also, water is better at heat dissipation due to the thermal efficiency of water being

25 times more than air, as long as the pool temperature is maintained at around 30°C. A lower temperature can increase the chances of shivering, while higher can make you sweat excessively.

Thus, exercise in water for periods over an hour should be complemented by a good hydration strategy, preferably maintaining body weight and water through regular drinking before, during and after exercise. Increased sweat production also increases the loss of electrolytes such as sodium and potassium. If you are going to be in the pool for more than 40–45 minutes it may be a good idea to consider an electrolyte-rich drink instead of water. Some sports drinks contain electrolytes but be mindful of their sugar content. Choose an isotonic drink where the composition mimics that of the blood rather than a hypertonic drink which has a high sugar content.

Water vs land-based exercise

Some elegant studies in the 1990s compared land-based exercises with water exercises in pregnant women at weeks 25 and 35.[10] The results suggest that heart rate and blood pressure were lower during the water-based exercise sessions. The study also found that due to the lower blood pressure, uterine blood flow was better maintained when swimming compared to cycling. However, exercise in the water increased urine production by about 200ml compared to land-based exercise at the same intensity.

Exercise in water allows for improved joint mobility. If you suffer from hypermobile joints either before or during pregnancy, then you need to be extra vigilant about your time in the water and consider modifying your session to reduce the hypermobility. Water acts as an analgesic too, so you may be unaware that you are extending your exercise beyond the healthy point if you do not pay attention to your joint movements.

I loved my aqua aerobics class. I enjoyed the bouncing around in the pool. It felt so comforting especially during the last days when everything else felt like a mountain climb. Twice a week I would do the aqua aerobics and alternated it with a bit of yoga and relaxation. To me it was a perfect mix of keeping active and staying relaxed.
Shruti

Impact of water exercises on your baby

Experiments studying the baby's response to immersion using detailed ultrasound data give us a fascinating insight into how babies cope in the uterus. In one study, after 20 minutes of exercise six out of seven foetuses had a slightly elevated heart rate when their mothers exercised on land, compared to only one when exercise was taken in the water.[11] However, all these elevated heart rates (tachycardia) were mild and transient with no reported long-term disadvantages for the babies.

In another experiment researchers looked at foetal urination from maternal exercise in water at 25 and 35 weeks and found that seven out of 11 babies showed increased urination after water exercise, and their bladder emptied and refilled again in the 20 minutes after exercise ended.[12] They found no adverse impact of increased urination by the foetus on their overall wellbeing. This experiment shows how immersion in water impacts the hormones that are responsible for regulating body water, and that these changes impact your baby's physiological response to your exercise.

Is swimming pool water safe?

Another concern many women may have is about the toxicity of the by-products of pool disinfectants. Many recent reports have suggested that pool disinfectant by-products are linked to disrupting human hormones. Reports of potential alterations in sperm quality and disruption to menstrual cycles have all been reported, in addition to potential links to certain cancers.

Swimming pools that are maintained to good hygiene standards still contain certain microbes and by-products of disinfectant materials like bromoform and chlorine. In addition, personal care products, sweat, urine, and faeces of swimmers, when mixed with these by-products, produce harmful substances such as halo benzoquinones that are implicated in hormonal disruption. Laboratory studies have shown the effects of these hormone disrupters at the gene and epigenetic levels.

Three large-scale studies have looked at swimming during pregnancy and the influence of pool water exposure on the foetus. The Danish National Birth Cohort study data from 1996–2002 on 74,486 pregnant women showed no impact from swimming for about 1.5 hours/week on birth weight or cleft palate.[13] Another large analysis, the UK-based Avon Longitudinal Parent and Child study in the 1990s, analysed 11,462 women and found that swimming regularly for up to one hour a week did not impact the birth weight of their infants.[14] However, the researchers did report a small negative association between swimming and the head circumference of the babies compared to the babies of women who did not exercise. An American study looking closely at changes in birth outcomes, including analysing infant umbilical cords for genetic level changes, also found this inverse association between head circumference and the time mothers spent in swimming pools.[15] The umbilical cords also showed high levels of erythroblasts (immature red blood cells) and low levels of a certain type of T-lymphoblast (CD4), which are cells that help coordinate the immune response. This indicates that the infants were physiologically responding to toxic exposure. However, none of these studies had any data about pool water, so these are rather generalised results.

Apopian and colleagues, who published data in 2013 from the massive National Birth Defect Prevention Study,[15] which collects data from 10 states across America, looking at 482,000 women, found no correlation between swimming pool exposure and 30 different kinds of birth defect.

With such large-scale data showing no adverse effects of pool disinfectant by-product exposure in pregnancy on infants, swimming throughout your pregnancy remains a safe activity with great potential benefits that compliment physical activity on land, due to the specific effects on joints and oedema.

Flexibility and mobility exercises

Keeping active during pregnancy can require a lot of motivation and inspiration. One way to keep up your activity levels is to add variety. Broadening out the way you use your body and being versatile with your movements will not only keep the boredom and lethargy at bay, but can also be an important way to keep your balance and mobility as your body changes.

Research comparing aerobic exercises and walking with flexibility-based exercises such as yoga shows that as pregnancy progresses these gentler forms of keeping active encourage more adherence (sticking) to exercise,[16–20] helping achieve an active lifestyle. Some studies have shown exercises such as Pilates, yoga and tai-chi to reduce the risks of falling, and to maintain core strength for moving and standing postures. These forms of exercises sit between aerobic and strength-training regimes, as they complement cardiovascular adaptations achieved during aerobic exercise and muscle and strength improvements from resistance training. Yoga and Pilates-type exercises tend to work on the functional capacity of the body and allow you to become fully aware of how to move with improved posture and core stability. This is most important during mid to late pregnancy when your physical shape changes most frequently.

The statistics indicate that almost 27% of pregnant women have taken a fall at some point in their pregnancy. This is pretty much the rate at which people tend to fall once they are over the age of 70. Thus, your changing anatomy, mechanics and hormonal laxity in ligaments and joints will have a big impact on your balance, flexibility and mobility. Studies have shown that women who participated in 12–20 weeks of yoga had significantly fewer falls compared to women who did not do any yoga.[20] Interestingly, the second trimester is when the risks of falling are greatest. There is about a 7kg increase in weight, and a 10cm increase in waist circumference between the second and third trimesters, and this almost sudden change is challenging to navigate for most women.

By your third trimester your balance may improve, but your walking speed tends to become significantly slower. Aerobic exercises will tend to feel a bit harder. You will find that postures in yoga and Pilates that are held for a short period allow you to reap the benefits of a strong practice when you can't get that from a relatively brisk walk.

Not all of us enjoy a run, swim or cycle ride, and neither do we all love weight training. So, obtaining all the physiological adaptations of the activities mentioned in the previous sections may feel cumbersome or boring. This is another reason our exercise needs to have breadth and variety. Modern yoga and Pilates classes tend to include strong physical postures that are held from a few seconds to a couple of minutes. The strength that comes from challenging our muscles and other tissues in this fashion, combined with the flow of movements over an hour or so, provides a perfect aerobic strength-based combination exercise that is less intense, more modifiable and perhaps more social than other forms. Studies have also shown that exercise classes such as yoga and Pilates create a more positive mindset and preparedness for birth, which is empowering.

> *I joined my pregnancy yoga class early in pregnancy (about 12 weeks) and honestly feel the benefits of regular, controlled pregnancy yoga have helped with all the usual aches and pains people talk about during pregnancy. I'm due any day now, and so many people have remarked on how well I get around and how much energy I have, and I'm about to be an 'older mum'! Other than the actual class itself, which is relaxing and pushes me to challenge my body's capabilities, the best thing has to be the sense of community I've found with all the ladies in the groups, It's a great way to make new friends and I've definitely made some friends for life through attending. It can be scary to join a new class, but I am glad I went along.* Natalie

One of the biggest advantages of yoga is that it provides a unique blend of breath modulation and physical movement.[21] This combination gives access to an opportunity to experience how our mindset can affect our physical abilities. The practice allows us to explore our physical limitations via a deeper mindful search of the true reasons behind our mental blocks or perceived obstructions. This combination of exploring our changing bodies and empowering our minds to reflect a positive experience of being pregnant can be truly transformational. Women who have previously not enjoyed being physically active have been able to slowly incorporate movement into their daily activities as they break down the barriers constructed by their own minds. This is particularly useful for birthing. Labour is physically demanding, and by being able to trust their physical abilities during pregnancy many women have been able to go into labour with a positive, more empowered mindset.

Exercises for mental resilience and emotional regulation

Pregnancy, birth and motherhood have their own unique stresses and anxieties which can be managed effectively so that we can feel positive antenatally and postnatally.

Until the 1990s stress and emotional distress were considered psychological issues and were treated as such in the majority of cases. However, thanks to sophisticated technology we now understand the nuanced interplay between hormones, emotions and behaviour and the subsequent impact on our wellbeing. Thus, behavioural elements of physical activity, rest and relaxation and modulations of breathing patterns are now the focus of many studies in improving mental health through mental resilience and emotional regulation.

Breath modulation is a powerful tool that can influence our other bodily functions in the short and long term. Deep slow breathing (DSB) has been used therapeutically for many years. Ancient sciences such as yoga, qigong and tai-chi all put great emphasis on breath modulation. Changes in our breathing display our immediate response to our environment. We hyperventilate when we are scared or angry, and slow our breathing down when we feel safe enough to rest. These simple messages sent via our breathing to the rest of the body impact every aspect of our physiology and more so when we are pregnant. They can affect your baby's physiology too. This continues into infancy and childhood, when you can influence your children's physiological responses to stress by co-regulating your breathing patterns with theirs and influencing their emotional regulation and long-term mental resilience.

Your response to your environment, interpreted via your breathing, is translated into a heart rate response (this is a function of the vagal nerve). When you are scared or angry and you hyperventilate, this message is taken to your autonomic nervous system (ANS), which activates the sympathetic nervous system (SNS) to increase your heart rate and release stress hormones like adrenaline and cortisol, which in turn increase your metabolism. All these physiological responses help you respond to the cause of your fear or anger. The opposite happens when you feel calm, protected and rested. The other arm of the ANS, the para-sympathetic nervous system (PsNS) tells your body to slow down and your heart rate and hormones respond by slowing down and decreasing your metabolic rate.

Your vagal nerve, which connects all major organs and bypasses the spinal cord, regulates your breathing with your heart rate. It does this on a breath-by-breath basis. When you inhale your heart rate goes up, and when you exhale your heart rate falls. The variation in the amount of rise and fall in your heart rate with every breath is a great marker of holistic wellbeing and is known as 'vagal tone'. The better the vagal tone, the more stress you can tolerate. It has been shown that people who are depressed tend to show very small variation in their vagal tone.

Interestingly, you can directly affect this tone. You can essentially train your body, via your breath modulation, to increase the tone of your vagal nerve. This makes you more resilient in terms of stress responses and allows you to temper your emotions.

Research in this area has been expanding steadily and from a variety of different types of research we now know that a breath rate of half your normal rate is what you need to aim for to begin seeing the benefits of improved tone of the vagal nerve. Most people at rest have a breath rate of 12–20 cycles per minute (cpm) at rest.[22] Some schools of thought, including advanced yoga practitioners, argue that a breath rate of 2–6 cycles per minute is needed to affect vagal tone. This is not that easy for a lot of us! A simple thing to start with is to take a few minutes each day to consciously reduce your breathing rate. Aim for fewer cycles of breath per minute for a few minutes at a time. Do what you can for as long as you can and it is comfortable for you. Start with a stop clock and lap your normal breath cycles for a minute. Do this on different days, at different times and after different activities. You will then see a general picture of your own breathing cycles. You may find some variations and it may vary depending on the stage of your pregnancy.

Next, start trying to exhale a bit longer in each cycle and see how that reduces your cycles per minute. Try to ignore your inhalation and just concentrate on extending your exhalation. Exhalation extension has multiple benefits compared to trying to slow both inhale and exhale. Extending exhalation helps with:

1. Reducing your breath cycles in a minute.
2. There is something called the sinus arrhythmia which is the increase in your heart rate when you inhale and a decrease in heart rate when you exhale. This means that

if you can extend your exhalation you will also be able to slow your heart rate.

3. The more pressure you can build in your lungs as you exhale the air out, the deeper you will be able to inhale, as the pressure inside your lungs will be greater than in the air around you. Therefore, as soon as you start to inhale and this pressure releases you will be able to bring in a lot more air into your lungs, creating a deeper, fuller inhalation.

The trick to slow, deep breathing, which is so therapeutic, is concentrating on extending your exhalations.

Another piece of the jigsaw in being able to improve your mental resilience is the element of relaxation added to deep breathing. A recent paper on pain management shows that deep breathing alone is not enough to decrease pain thresholds.[23] However, when combined with relaxation, deep breathing is very effective in reducing pain thresholds. You can use this breath modulation practice in conjunction with other relaxation techniques, such as in a bath, or even using it to initiate relaxation at the end of the day before bed. This is also great for improving your sleep.

The same study found that people who paid too much attention to their breathing did not benefit as much as people who seemed more relaxed about it. This is a reminder that breath modulation exercises need to be practised regularly to really see how powerful they can be in reducing stress and anxiety. Regularity is the key, not the amount of time you spend. You can increase the time eventually if you feel you enjoy it.

We were trying for a baby for three years and, after two losses, this pregnancy felt like every day I was walking on eggshells. I would be really excited one moment and the next would become super anxious. Since I had another six weeks before we could get a scan, if I had carried on like that, I am pretty sure I would have driven my partner mad. My partner is a calm person by nature but not me, I needed to manage my anxiety but I didn't really talk about it to anyone. A friend of mine suggested meditation and I laughed that I couldn't even sit still for half a minute, no way would I be able to meditate. I started yoga instead. What I didn't realise was that all that breathing practice in yoga had started to help me. I didn't even know it till my partner pointed it out. I don't think I would have attended the class if it was meditation, but because it wasn't called that somehow it made it accessible for me. Anabelle

If you have heard that meditation helps calm the mind, but you always found it hard to do, or to stick to, the breath modulation practice is a gateway to developing some meditative elements in your day. As you get comfortable exercising your breath you will be able to get into deeper aspects of meditation. For the breath-based exercise, you do not need incense burning, or a special place that is serene – you don't even need to sit down. Just start wherever you are, by slowing and extending your exhalations, slowly get a rhythm and then come back to it another day. One technique I have used with clients is borrowed from Jerry Seinfeld's habit of writing a joke a day. Just come to your breath awareness each day, no matter when or where. That's it. You just have to turn up. Mark an X on the calendar when you do… and try not breaking the chain.

In the next chapter I will detail some simple tips and solutions I have used both in my own practice and professionally that will help you make physical activity a sustainable part of your lifestyle, not just something you do during pregnancy and postnatally.

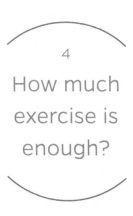

4

How much exercise is enough?

Time is not equal to impact

The first important aspect of physical activity is to remember that you do not need to do a lot in one session. Think about being *less sedentary* rather than worrying about incorporating yet another activity into your tight schedule. The trick is to consider very small changes to your current lifestyle that will prevent you from sitting down for extended periods. This could include simple things like making sure the kettle is a bit of a walk away. You could also use technology, such as alarms or activity trackers, to prompt you to move.

Goals are for losers

If you are thinking of doing more exercise, it is important you don't start big. In fact, research has consistently shown that a 'goal' orientated approach has short-term effects. What I mean by that is not that the motivation that comes from having goals is invalid, but that it can mean you adopt short-term approaches that do not get incorporated deep into your way of living. If you want to be active for the rest of your life, starting at this amazingly important time in your life, you need something stronger and deeper than an event or a date-oriented goal.

If you use a goal-based approach you may become more active before and/or during pregnancy, but as soon as that motivation has gone, once you've had your baby, you will find yourself reverting to your old habits. After more than 20 years of working with a variety of people, from elite athletes to people who want to manage their weight, I have found that whatever 'strategies' you may employ to be more active, the only ones that have a long-term impact are the ones that get incorporated into your everyday lifestyle.

A goal-based approach makes your mind focus on the end date/event, after which you have already (even unconsciously) given your mind permission to relax. You constantly find yourself thinking about the end point, imagining achieving your goal and feeling like a winner. There is no plan for afterwards, other than moving to another goal. Perhaps you start exercising when you start trying for a baby and feel like you have achieved your goal when you get pregnant. You may then have to set a different goal to be active during pregnancy. Then after the baby is born you may set a goal for some postnatal weight loss or strength-building, which may motivate you till you have lost those extra pounds… but what next? You will have to keep finding these glittery prizes in the distance and you will always be moving from one trophy to the next. Each time you will need to find fresh reasons to be and stay active. This constant search is not only tiring, but can also lead to you taking drastic measures if you perceive one goal is more urgent than another. This is the dreaded yo-yo. Yo-yo is not really about losing and gaining weight; it's gaining motivation and losing motivation.

I am convinced that anyone can be active, lose weight, climb mountains and run ultra-marathons if they are motivated. But a healthy life comes from doing the things you need to do even when your motivation is at its lowest point. This the root of the problem with a goal-orientated approach. Most people are very motivated at the start when they set the goal, but as time goes by and the novelty wears off it becomes harder and harder to motivate yourself to keep up the efforts. Research has shown that the further away you are from the initial goal, the more dedication, effort and resilience you will need to bring to the task in order to keep up the same level of motivation.

This makes complete sense, but my view is why take the hard way when there is a smaller, simpler road, not littered with trophies and accolades. This is the imperceptible chain of everyday activities. It's more an alleyway than a road. No passers-by, no cheerleaders and certainly no trophies... but once you get used to it you won't need them. It's a bit like how you feel when you brush your teeth. Do you need motivation to brush your teeth? The prize is not 'visible', there is no clear goal, but for most of our lives we brush our teeth morning and night without ever questioning our efforts. In the same way, not sitting down for extended periods (more than 20–30 minutes at a time) should simply feel uncomfortable – like not brushing your teeth. The prize is not only your health, mobility and freedom from aches, but also a legacy of a healthy lifestyle for your children.

Getting the most out of your activity patterns

Physical activity is the sum total of frequency (F), intensity (I), duration/time (T) and mode (M) of your physical movements. You do not need to spend more time being active to get more out of it. There are other ways to improve your fitness than just going for an hour's walk. For example, you can increase the *intensity* of the exercise when you have less *time* (duration) or fewer free days (frequency). It is the overall effect that counts. Knowing this allows you to keep active without having to compromise your lifestyle or exercise on days when you don't feel up to it. The trick is to create a habit of thinking and consciously incorporating physical activity within your day so that it is no longer something you need to carve out time for.

You can modify your exercise by changing the frequency, intensity and time (FIT). As you get used to moving more, you will notice that each week you can manage a certain number of days or an average frequency (F) of some sort of exercise programme. As you establish the frequency, then on a daily basis you can determine how much or how little time (T) you have on that particular day. You can choose to increase intensity (I) if you have less time, or take it slow if you have more. Finally, based on the frequency, intensity and time modifications you can choose the mode (M) of exercise. Could you do some quick weights on a high-intensity less time day, or could you go for a lovely park walk on a low-intensity more time day? This is the principle of FIT-M movement. Even though FIT-M is not much different from the popular FITT (Frequency, Intensity, Time, Type) principle, it is a fundamental shift in the way you prioritise your physical activity.

The FIT-M principle gives you a clear order for which aspect of your exercise you should plan first and why.

1. Plan your 'frequency' first. Once you know the number of times you can fit in moving more each week you can look at the specifics of each session.
2. For each session, you can ask: 'How long do I have

today?' This will help you determine the *time* which will automatically answer the question of *intensity*:

- More time – low intensity
- Less time – high intensity

Remember both are important to incorporate.

3. Depending on whether you are going to do a high or low-intensity exercise session you can choose your *mode*. If it is a high-intensity session you can choose weights or a strong yoga or Pilates practice that doesn't last long but includes strength and agility. On a low-intensity day you can choose a slow flow yoga session or a lovely swim or a long walk in the park with friends.

Slowly aim to move more often, by a small amount every day. You can play around with FIT-M and get an overall incremental benefit of physical activity which will shield you against the health risks of staying sedentary. I am highlighting the *lifetime* effect of physical activity here, rather than focusing on the narrow time frame of pregnancy and the postnatal period, because committing to physical activity as part of life will normalise it during the perinatal period too. But in later chapters we will see that there are some very specific reasons why physical activity is especially important during pregnancy and postnatally, which will hopefully inspire you further.

Understanding the progressive overload principle

Once you build up your exercise habit and your body is used to moving more and not tolerating long periods of sitting, you will soon realise that you feel better. To reap the big rewards you can now start to think about how to maximise the time you exercise to gain all the health benefits of exercise for your pregnancy, birth and the postnatal period, even passing on the benefits to your unborn baby.

Thinking about the progressive overload principle will allow you to increase your levels of activity without having to compromise on your lifestyle. Progressive overload simply means that you need to make your exercise a tiny bit harder than the last time to stay strong and get stronger. Your body soon adapts to the level of stress and demand you put on it. During pregnancy this happens almost automatically as we get bigger and heavier: if you keep your exercise exertion levels the same, particularly in resistance exercise involving the lower body such as squats, lunges and even walking, you will get stronger.

There is no reason why you can't change aspects of your training to get a higher exertion level. You can increase the time you spend walking or swimming, or make it a bit faster. When you are doing any resistance-based exercise with weights or bands, increase the repetitions instead of increasing the load (weights). When you are short of time, increase the resistance and keep the repetitions the same.

By playing with FIT-M you will be able to keep active without making a big fuss about physical activity in your life. This will let you relax and enjoy moving your body rather than focussing on specific things and goals that can sometimes be counterproductive to enjoyment. You are only likely to stick with something if it becomes enjoyable and non-demanding, and you don't need masses of motivation to get you to do it. Remember this is just a principle; you don't need to get too bogged down by it in every session. The general trend is what matters.

Wrapping women in cotton wool

One myth that simply won't go away is that pregnant women should 'take it easy'. This is fine when you are feeling unwell, or suffering from the physical onslaught of pregnancy, IVF or a new baby. If you are tired, then the most prudent thing to do is ignore all calls to exercise and *rest*. Research is very clear on the importance of rest and recovery over exercise. However, this need for rest must be determined by you and you alone. Don't let external voices who believe you should rest through the first trimester (without good medical reason) convince you to lead a sedentary life. Studies have shown that women who exercise before and in early pregnancy (before 20 weeks) get the benefits of this exercise throughout the rest of their pregnancies, and their birth outcomes improve (see Chapter 6).[1,2]

When the foetus is developing organs and organ systems, physical activity has been shown to protect against excessive free radical damage that correlates to reduced placental function and increased miscarriage rates. Foetal and placental growth is enhanced in women who are adapted to exercise, which in turn brings better functional capacity of the placenta to allow for increased oxygen and nutrient delivery.[3] Your body can do this while also fulfilling your need for increased blood flow into your muscles. There is no evidence to support the idea that your exercise somehow compromises the development and growth of your baby in the first trimester.

Exercise classes and teacher-training programmes for pregnancy exercise all advocate starting classes or exercise regimes in the second trimester, despite evidence suggesting very low risk of exercise to both mother and baby in the first trimester. This sort of advice is based on a lack of knowledge of the current evidence, and fear of litigation.

Practical ways to increase your physical activity:

1. Reduce the time you spend sitting down. Have an alarm set to remind you get up from your desk or sofa after 30–40 minutes. It is easy to forget how long we have been sitting down for. Walk and move for at least a few minutes before sitting down again. Line up chores that you can do throughout your day for your time off the sofa.

2. When the weather is good get some fresh air and go outside. You can do whatever you prefer. If the activity involves squatting, bending and carrying stuff then even better, as it activates your big muscle groups.

3. Join a specialist pregnancy exercise group. It will help you commit to some exercise, make friends and keep up your motivation. Make sure you pick a time of the day when you are most likely to go, both time and energy-wise.

4. Make it social. Even if you are going out on your own, arrange to have coffee/lunch with friends or family after your exercise. This will motivate you not to cancel your exercise. Choose a place where you can show up in exercise clothes!

5. Take care of your mental health through physical activity. Using breath modulation and meditation-based principles will make it easier to manage stress, anxiety and general worry.

6. If you are using your local gym and have been using weights before pregnancy do not stop when you get pregnant. Modify your exercises to keep your intensity at moderate levels. Don't pick weights that are so heavy you can do fewer than 10 repetitions. You should comfortably be able to do 15–20 repetitions for each exercise and not be completely out of breath. A small

amount of hyperventilation for 30–60 seconds can be tolerated if you rest after the set to completely eliminate any shortness of breath before the next set.

7. The ability to maintain full sentences when you talk during aerobic exercises such as walking, swimming and cycling is a good measure of moderate intensity.

8. A simple rule of thumb, without getting into calculating heart rates and heart rate reserves, is not to push yourself so that you can't talk comfortably and are hyperventilating.

9. Aim to get some variety into your exercise programme. Add flexibility, mobility and core-strengthening exercises to your mix.

10. Aim to get three to five active sessions of 30–50 minutes in a week. Public Health England has a simple 150 minute/ week guidance that is a good measure.

11. Keep hydrated throughout the day (again alarm prompts can work well) and eat a healthy snack about 30–60 minutes before exercise and a good meal after.

12. If you are on medications, make a specific exercise plan with your GP/midwife or qualified exercise specialist and keep a record of your activities with any change in symptoms or your wellbeing. Review this plan regularly or when you think necessary.

Environmental considerations
Heat stress

What do we know about exercising in hot and humid conditions? There is patchy new and emerging research that suggests our old fears about hot environments causing birth defects might not be fully justified.

In the 1960s Dr Marshall Edwards conducted a series of interesting experiments that have been used as seminal evidence in this field.[4–6] He exposed pregnant guinea pigs to about an hour of heat at 42–43°C. The young of these mothers displayed deficits in brain function and reduced brain size. In addition, there were other consequences including foetal resorption (loss of pregnancy), general growth retardation of the young and developmental defects. In particular anencephaly (the absence of major parts of the brain, skull or scalp) was attributed to heat stress.

These studies led to the publication of other studies in humans, particularly looking at fever and brain defects, which showed that maternal core temperatures of over 39°C or an increase in core temperature of ~1.0–2.0°C led to an increased risk of developmental toxicity in early pregnancy.

An interesting Finnish letter in the *BMJ* in 1979 considered the popularity of the use of sauna in Finland and reported a small study showing that 100 pregnant women who continued the use of sauna (70–100°F for 10–30 minutes) in pregnancy did not have babies with congenital malformations, including anencephaly (0.32/1,000 births in Finland, which is no different to the number of babies born to women who did not use sauna).[7]

It is important to note that a core body temperature in pregnant women of more than 39°C has been long considered the critical threshold for teratogenic toxicity. But current guidelines are not specific about exercise or exposure to heat and humidity. Moreover, individual interpretations and altered perception of heat in pregnancy can all increase the vagueness of the guidelines and may lead to undue stress when you exercise on a hot day.

Then there is the whole issue of measuring core temperature. This is a very hard thing to do for regular people exercising, as thermometers generally measure skin temperature, which is different from core temperature. How would you know that your core temperature has risen to a critical threshold? This is really a question for the laboratory/academia.

At rest your unborn baby's temperature is higher than your body's and during exercise it is the other way around. Heat transfer during pregnancy takes place via the placental wall and uterine blood flow. Therefore, reduced blood flow to the baby can be protective for your baby, by not letting his core temperature rise with yours.

Pregnancy is also a time when your thermoregulatory capacity is enhanced significantly and thus as your pregnancy progresses temperature rises are slower. One of the reasons for this is that as you get bigger, you have a higher surface area, so heat dissipates faster. Therefore, the same amount of exercise intensity does not create the same increase in core body temperature.

The current evidence from systematic reviews and meta-analyses shows that even when pregnant women exercised for 20–30 minutes at intensities of 80–90% of their maximal heart rate throughout their pregnancies their core temperature did not exceed 38°C.[8] This suggests that there is a low risk of your core temperature rising to 39°C while doing moderate to high intensity exercise up to 90% of your maximal capacity for up to 35 minutes at ambient temperatures of 25°C and 45% relative humidity.

Exercising in water has further protective effects on rise in core temperature as water has approximately 25 times the thermal conductivity of air. Also, water decreases cardiac strain by facilitating increased cardiac filling (more blood in the heart before pumping), which in turn keeps the heart rate low and core temperature rises more slowly. Water-based activities can thus be maintained for 20–45 minutes as opposed to 35 minutes on land.

Saunas at 70°C at 15% relative humidity and warm baths

at 40°C can both be enjoyed for up to 20 minutes before core temperature starts to inch towards 38°C.

No studies that have ever recorded core temperature rises with physical activity beyond 38°C, a whole degree lower than the 39°C teratogenic threshold which may cause developmental toxicity.

Surface

It is important to protect against falls as they are unpredictable and we don't know how we are going to land and what impact that will have on the uterus. It is the physical insult to the body that we want to avoid.

Exercising on softer surfaces such as grass, carpeted floors, snow and sandy beaches allows for better shock absorption of any high-intensity impact, but at the same time challenges balance. So unless you are used to these surfaces before and during your whole pregnancy, so small changes to your centre of gravity can be controlled due to constant practice, do not start exercising on these surfaces midway through your pregnancy.

Hard surfaces such as tarmac, concrete floors and pavements can increase the force that is passed through your joints, especially if you run. This force can cause micro-tears in the ligaments and cartilage or even flare up old injuries. If joints are laxer, or there is increased mobility, the force can be even more impactful. Sometimes small injuries or latent problems can resurface in the postnatal period.

Surfaces with inclines and declines should be navigated with great attention, even if they are familiar paths. The change in your base of support and centre of mass throughout pregnancy can throw up unexpected challenges even on well-known routes.

Water and other weight-bearing surfaces not only have a

soothing impact on the strains of the body, but also help with balancing and movement.

One of the most important surfaces to be mindful of is winter roads and pavements covered in sleet and ice. These slippery surfaces are unpredictable and it is easy to lose balance.

Clothing

Clothing in pregnancy can be tricky in general, without getting into exercise clothes. You may struggle to find appropriate clothing even in the early days. However, there is now specific maternity active wear that can be made from great technical material. Here are a few considerations when choosing exercise clothes:

- Allow yourself to be comfortable and avoid very tight-fitting clothes in which you may feel restricted. Sometimes tightness in your clothing could be just because of your changing body proportions.
- A great way to achieve less sedentary behaviour is to have comfortable clothes you can stretch and move in throughout your day, eliminating any need for special 'exercise' clothes, unless you are doing special activities like swimming.
- Heat dissipation should also be a consideration, so choose clothes that do not make you feel hot too easily. Dressing in a multitude of thin layers that can be removed or put back on easily is a great way to keep cool and comfortable when you exercise.
- Bras need to be structured, comfortable and secure so that the delicate and changing tissues in your breasts are well cared for.
- Shoes need to be comfortable, fitted correctly and airy

to allow for transfer of heat. If you have any pelvic girdle pain or other orthopaedic considerations, get specialist advice and gait analysis to make sure you are not letting footwear cause your posture or movement to have a negative impact on your body.

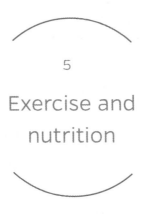

5

Exercise and nutrition

Hydration first

Becoming pregnant will increase your need for water for normal functioning within 6–8 weeks of conception. As your blood volume increases the need for fluids increases too. If there is not enough fluid to maintain this blood volume it can put the cardiovascular system under considerable strain, increasing blood pressure and in certain cases beginning a cascade of physiological events that may lead to hypertension and pre-eclampsia. Studies have shown that women with hypertension have less total body water and are thus at a greater risk of dehydration.

Lack of enough liquids in the diet places more strain on the renal system, affecting the kidneys under strain. With increased energy and nutrient requirements, the kidneys work harder during pregnancy. Your water intake will also influence your weight gain during pregnancy. Research indicates that people without optimum hydration are at a greater risk of developing obesity.[1] Insufficient total body water has been shown to increase the risk of low birth weight infants and premature births.[2]

If you exercise during pregnancy, you need to be even more vigilant about your fluid intake. Your breathing is more laboured in pregnancy, and you tend to lose more water through your breath, which is exacerbated by exercise. Core body temperature is maintained via increased sweating, and with a larger surface area as you get bigger you tend to sweat more than normal during exercise while pregnant.

Do not wait to drink till you are thirsty. By the time you feel and recognise thirst, you are already on your way to being dehydrated. A good general strategy for fluid is little and often. Don't force yourself to drink a lot of water at once if you think you have forgotten to drink for a while.

I had a sticky note that said 'water' on my desk at work, beside my bed and randomly dotted across the house. I had a small water bottle next to the note. I have used this trick for years and every time I read the note, the water is right there for me to drink! Debbie

After exercise, it is important to pay attention to your thirst as this will help you to continue to regain any lost fluids. It can take more than a couple of days to completely replenish fluid reserves. So if you have done more vigorous exercise one day, go easy on the next and continue to pay attention to your water intake. You can also count tea and coffee (in moderation) as part of your fluids. If your coffee is not a strong espresso-style drink, the water and milk you add to it will go towards building your hydration status. Also, foods high in water like fruits and leafy vegetables, and meals like broths and soups count towards your fluid intake. Be wary of sports drinks with their high sugar content. If possible, stick to water or diluted fruit juices, avoiding artificial sweeteners.

Keep a look out for the tell-tale signs of dehydration throughout your pregnancy. These include reduced trips to the bathroom, darker urine than normal, dry eyes and headaches and dizziness.

Fluid intake for breastfeeding mothers

There is surprisingly little research into fluid intake and breastmilk production. A Cochrane review concluded that there was little evidence about fluid intake and milk production in lactating women.[3] So what we know about the combined implications of breastfeeding and exercise on the hydration of both mother and baby and milk production is extrapolated from various research ideas, including studies looking at women living in deserts, women breastfeeding during fasting and even other mammals such as cows, goats and camels.

We do know that infants are susceptible to dehydration due to their large surface area, which increases sweating, and their underdeveloped renal system that cannot modulate urine composition to conserve water. However, infants can regulate breastfeeding frequency to match their hydration needs. So they tend to feed more often when it's hot or when mum is dehydrated.

Both anecdotal and some extrapolated data seems to suggest that women produce on average 700–800ml of breastmilk over a 24-hour period, and lactating mothers tend to drink 1,000ml more than their non-pregnant, non-lactating counterparts. This shows that without conscious effort mothers tend to consume the extra fluids they need to produce milk. Breastfeeding itself promotes a powerful thirst stimulus, which may be due to the high prolactin secretion around the time of suckling, which is why you may have noticed that as soon as your baby starts to suckle you feel thirsty! Prolactin is also increased when we exercise, particularly in the heat. Thus it seems that the role of prolactin in stimulating thirst is broader than just breastfeeding. However, we do not know much about prolactin status in lactating and exercising mothers. We do not know if this combination makes mothers more susceptible to dehydration, or whether the role of prolactin ensures that the hydration status of both baby and mother is maintained.

Women who live in hot conditions show that milk production is remarkably resilient and short-term reduced fluid intake doesn't lead to obvious dehydration in either baby or mother. This is possibly due to subconscious behavioural changes, such as engaging in short-term hyper-hydration strategies (drinking a lot of water when possible before going through a period of reduced water intake). There is very little evidence on how effective these are.

If you are exercising and breastfeeding, try to be more vigilant about your fluid intake. Carry water with you whenever possible, drink often and don't wait to feel parched. Moderate to intense exercise sessions, especially in hot and humid conditions for more than 20 minutes, may lead to a reduction in body water that can take 24–48 hours to replenish – and longer if you are exclusively breastfeeding. So be mindful about consecutive exercise sessions in the heat, or high-intensity sessions, as they will eventually lead to chronic dehydration if you cannot replenish that water between sessions.

Watch out for signs of dehydration in both you and your baby. Reduced urine output, darker than usual urine, parched throat, headaches and dizziness are all indicators. Babies tend to deteriorate quickly when dehydrated. Take them to the GP or hospital if you notice any of the signs of dehydration, such as seeming drowsy, breathing fast, few or no tears when they cry, a soft spot on their head that sinks inwards (sunken fontanelle), dry mouth, dark yellow pee or have not had a pee in the last 12 hours, or cold and blotchy-looking hands and feet.

The basics of nutrition in relation to exercise

Energy requirements during pregnancy

There are considerable individual variations in energy expenditure and intake among pregnant women. Most research data indicate that the energy requirements of pregnant women range from 2,000–3,000kcal/day, which is not substantially higher than non-pregnant women. This means on average you need just under 200kcal extra per day, in your third trimester only. Your basal metabolic rate (the amount of energy you need to simply survive) is only 5% higher in your first trimester, 10% higher by mid pregnancy and 25% more in your third trimester. If you were within the normal BMI (20–25) category and were active before you got pregnant, you may not need to increase your energy intake in the first two trimesters. Your body and your diet will be well adjusted to your activity levels. However, if you were dieting to lose weight before becoming pregnant, you will probably want to return to your pre-dieting energy intake.

There is no need to 'eat for two'. Your energy intake is sufficient for all your baby's needs. Your digestive system adapts to be able to absorb more nutrients from your food and your placenta becomes more efficient in transporting these nutrients to your baby. Your body can identify which nutrients are required at any given time for your baby's growth and you can upregulate the intake, absorption and transport of specific nutrients accordingly.

If you get your energy intake from a wide variety of foods, you can rest assured that you are most likely going to meet your vitamin and mineral requirements too. Most guidance indicates that apart from specific nutrients such as folic acid there is very little evidence for the need for extra nutrient supplements during pregnancy. However, this only applies if you have a high quality, varied diet. There is no evidence that supplementation of vitamins and minerals at a moderate level (not excessive doses) does long-term harm. However, there is evidence of moderate quality that shows no benefit from supplementation.[4] Seek individualised advice from a registered nutritionist or dietitian for your specific needs if you are concerned.

When you exercise during pregnancy you may find that your appetite temporarily increases until your body can regulate the energy intake and expenditure over a longer period. It is important to listen to your body and eat healthy foods if you feel like eating more.

Macronutrients: carbohydrates, fats and protein
Carbohydrates
Exercise and physical activity help alter body composition by increasing lean tissue and decreasing fat storage. Lean tissue is metabolically very demanding, in that it requires more energy to retain lean tissue than fat. Therefore, exercise and the right nutrients are equally important when it comes to maintaining good body composition.

During pregnancy, our hormones adapt towards more energy-saving routes to protect the survival of the foetus and ensure adequate fat storage for feeding after birth. Insulin, the hormone which regulates the carbohydrates we eat, acts less readily, to allow carbohydrates to be driven to the placenta instead of being used as energy for the mother. Our liver increases production of carbohydrates, which ensures a constant supply for the baby even if the mother does not eat often. So, when you exercise at moderate to high intensity, and your body wants to predominately use carbohydrate as a source of energy, you will need to make sure you eat adequate carbohydrates to ensure your physical needs are met despite the shift in hormonal conditions.

You may find that after exercise (sometimes after a few weeks of exercising regularly) you crave carbohydrate-rich foods. This is normal and it is important that you consume carbohydrates that are complex to digest and not simple sugars that will make your insulin overactive and cause harm in the long run. A series of experiments by James Clapp in the 1990s elegantly showed the impact of the type of carbohydrates eaten by pregnant women on infant birth weight.[5] Simple carbohydrates like white bread, white pasta and added sugars such as glucose-fructose syrups in ready meals and snacks all contribute to reduced insulin insensitivity and development of GDM. They also encourage your baby's system to develop lower insulin sensitivity and thus increases their risk of developing type-2 diabetes. These risks were mitigated if women consumed more fibre, and more complex carbohydrates such as bran bread or whole wheat pasta.

One good way to dampen the insulin spike after meals is to mix carbohydrates with fat or protein. Fat and protein are both very hard to digest, so if you butter your white toast, the simple carbohydrate (sugars) from the toast is mixed with the fat from the butter making the sugar release more slowly into your bloodstream. The speed at which carbohydrates enter the bloodstream from your gut is what matters most when it comes to insulin response. This is important as part of a long-term diet strategy to prevent diabetes, weight gain and other metabolic disturbances. Eating protein with the carbohydrates has the same effect. So, if you are using white pasta, adding some fish, chicken or tofu will help slow down the sugar release from the gut into your blood.

Fats

Dietary fat is not the same as body fat. We can make body fat from any energy source: it is a way the body stores excess energy to be used in times of decreased intake, such as famine, or when we need more energy than we may be able to consume, such as during lactation. During pregnancy, our bodies get more efficient at storing excess energy and thus make it harder to use fat as source of energy too.

Certain fats, such as long-chain fatty acids found in fish oils that are essential in the diet, are particularly important for foetal brain development and other tissues such as the retina. The need for essential fatty acids is greatest in third trimester when the brain grows rapidly.

There is increasing evidence of the role of essential fatty acids in helping exercise efforts by regulating appetite, increasing the use of fat as an energy source, repairing tissues and reducing DOMS (delayed onset muscular soreness). Thus, not only are the essential fatty acids important for foetal development, but they will also support your exercise programme.

Protein

Most adult women are recommended to consume about 45g/day (0.6g/kg of body weight) of protein. Protein requirement in pregnancy increases within weeks of becoming pregnant. The government guidelines (SACN) recommend additional protein intake of about 6g/day (0.88g/kg of body weight) to support increased tissue production, such as the placenta, and the growth needs of the foetus.

Some studies have shown an additional need for protein if you exercise, but this is controversial, as exercise adaptations make your body more efficient at protein absorption and use. In addition, exercise protects your muscles and other lean tissues against breakdown, reducing the need to constantly build them up.

Exercise nutrition principles

There are some simple rules worth remembering when you exercise during pregnancy (or for that matter at any point in your life):

1. *Try not to do moderate to high intensity exercise on an empty stomach. Eat a small snack rich in complex carbohydrates and a small amount of protein (like nut butter or a nut-based drink) at least 30–40 minutes beforehand.*

   High-intensity exercise (where you can't speak in full sentences) has no adverse effects on your pregnancy or baby if you keep it under 90% of your maximal capacity. But this level of exercise cannot readily use fat as a source of energy and you will need to rely on stored carbohydrates in your muscles to supply energy. This is because fat takes at least 20 minutes or so to be mobilised from the tissues and trickle into your blood, which is then dispersed to the exercising muscles. At a higher intensity muscles rely on 'local' energy stores, which is carbohydrates (glycogen) stored in the muscles themselves. If you make sure there is a constant supply of carbohydrates from both the muscles (stored previously from the food you have eaten over 24–48 hours) and the blood (from the digestion of pre-exercise snack) you will 'spare' your protein, which can be used for repair and growth rather than be broken down for energy.

2. *Low intensity exercise can be done on a fairly empty stomach to encourage fat-burning.*

   However, if you have any symptoms of hypoglycaemia (low blood sugar levels, dizziness, light-headedness) eat a small snack 30 minutes before exercising.

   This is not a recommendation for fasting during pregnancy. It is just a simple way to enhance fat use as a source of energy when you are doing low intensity exercise (exercise under 50% of your maximal capacity). This level of exercise does not require large amounts of energy in short periods of time. Your body can match your energy requirements with the slow release of fat from your tissues. Mostly healthy individuals, including pregnant women, can exercise for about 30 minutes or so (slowly build up to this time if you need to) despite not having eaten for a couple of hours. Our ancestors did not have vending machines and corner stores, and we have evolved to survive periods of low food intake without difficulty.

   However, if you have been active before pregnancy and perhaps done low-intensity exercise on an empty stomach after an overnight fast, it may be worth adding a small pre-exercise snack while you are pregnant. Pregnancy hormones induce insulin resistance, so you may feel mildly hypoglycaemic despite being used to exercising on an empty stomach. This is a time to listen to your body, not stick to your old habits. Subtle changes to your nutrition strategy will ensure you can keep up your fitness levels.

3. *Always make sure you have a non-sugar drink with you and don't wait till you get thirsty to drink.*

   As we have seen, pregnancy is a time to ensure you do not get chronically dehydrated, which could increase your risk of hyperthermia (increase in core body temperature) that will slow or shut down vital functions in your body and compromise your baby's growth. Exercise in hot and humid climates, even high-intensity exercise, is well tolerated in fit and adapted pregnant women if they can maintain blood volume, electrolyte composition and blood sugar levels. For all these essential functions it is imperative that you pay attention to hydration.

If you are going to do any exercise for more than an hour, consider an electrolyte-based drink to replenish any lost minerals in sweat. But choose a drink that is low in sugar (isotonic drinks are better than hypertonic drinks) as you can replenish sugars at your meal after exercise.

4. *Eat as soon as you can after you finish exercise.*
   This will ensure you replenish nutrients from your diet, rather than your body breaking down tissues to maintain a continuous supply of nutrients to your baby. Pregnancy hormones allow your body to absorb more nutrients from your diet than normal. This is one of the reasons why your requirements do not increase dramatically. Your body is even more efficient in nutrient transfer after exercise as your muscles are depleted and amplify their nutrient absorption capacity. Take advantage of this heightened period of super-absorption of nutrients and make sure you get a good dose of healthy fats, carbohydrates and protein after exercise.

5. *After exercise, try eating a mixture of complex carbohydrates like oats or bran bread or nuts to ensure a constant slow supply of sugars in your bloodstream.*
   The simpler the carbohydrates, the less digestion they need to be absorbed. Simple sugars from our gut enter the blood easily. This stimulates the production of insulin, as anything above normal sugar levels needs 'clearing' away from the blood. If you eat a piece of white bread, which is

easily digested as it has no fibre to delay the sugars entering the blood, the sugars will flood the bloodstream and more insulin will be required to clear the blood of the excess sugars. But if you eat a piece of bran bread the fibre stops the quick release of sugars into your blood, reducing the insulin response. This means the sugars enter your blood more slowly, providing a constant supply of energy over a long period of time. This also helps replenish your stores of glycogen.

6. *Avoid going hungry for very long periods (more than four hours at a time).*

   Our bodies respond very differently to long-term fasting, such as more than four hours without food. Energy use shifts from mixed sources of carbohydrates and fat to more fat and protein. Protein is the only source of nitrogen for our bodies, which is essential for every single process. Thus, using protein as a source of energy (through the breakdown of lean tissue) deprives our system of growth and repair molecules (amino acids). It is also hard to build lean tissue back up.

7. *Try and eat some protein, such as lean meat or nuts, at every meal to ensure that you maintain the growth of your baby and meet your own needs.*

   Physical activity increases the need for protein in addition to the extra needs of pregnancy. Protein cannot be digested in huge amounts at the same time. Thus, it is essential to eat protein more often during the day rather than having one big protein meal. Adding small amounts of protein will also help reduce the insulin response to carbohydrates in your meals.

8. *Variety is a great way to ensure you meet your vitamin and mineral needs in addition to your energy needs.*

   Try to include at least three to five different colours on your plate. Most foods derive their colour from their vitamin content. Meeting your vitamin and mineral needs is what alerts the brain to make you feel full. The assumption is that, by the time you have eaten enough vitamins and minerals, which are needed in small quantities, you will have consumed enough energy. This is the reason that fast foods that are low in vitamins and minerals can be consumed in high amounts. It is easy to overeat because your brain does not register fullness due to the lack of vitamins and minerals in the meal.

9. *Do not cut down on food during pregnancy and maintain at least 2,000–3,000kcal/day of energy intake.*
   Pregnancy is definitely not a time to cut down on calories or to be on a diet, especially if you are thinking of being active during your pregnancy. Although there are no additional energy needs until the third trimester, it is still important to meet your normal daily requirements to support your pregnancy and grow your baby.

All the above points are general strategies to support your exercise efforts. However, it is really important to take individualised advice and guidance from a suitably qualified professional if needed.

Gut health and the microbiome

There are around 100 trillion bacteria in your gut, and the ratio of human cells to bacteria in our bodies is close to 1:1. Each person's particular mix of bacteria is unique, and starts to form while they are still in the womb. Later, the microbiome is influenced by mode of birth, environmental exposures such as maternal antibiotic use before and during pregnancy, and major illness, and it can affect your health throughout your life. Gut bacteria digest indigestible particles in your food, releasing important nutrients into your system.

When you are pregnant, the composition of your microbiome can have an impact on the birth of your baby and their long-term health. Women with more favourable bacterial colonies in their gut tend to have better outcomes.

The anti-inflammatory properties of the bacteria protect the foetus from rejection at the placental bed. Research shows that women who suffer from premature rupture of membranes have less favourable gut microbiota.[6] Also, women with high BMI, GDM and leaky gut syndrome also tend to have altered microbiota compared to women without these conditions.

The gut-brain axis

There is a two-way relationship between our guts and our brains. Normal brain development and functioning relies on a healthy gut. There is an information highway from the gut to the brain via the vagus nerve and information from the brain flows constantly to the gut via hormones. If this relationship works well, our brains can respond to threats from the external environment through gut health. For example, if you are experiencing stress, stress hormones such as cortisol increase inflammation in the gut, changing the gut microbiota. This change is then reflected in brain activity and can influence our behavioural response to stress.

The maternal gut-brain axis is an important part of brain development during foetal life. It is becoming an important focus for research looking at the connections between brain neurochemistry and emotional and behavioural responses in individuals. For example, conditions such as autism have been linked to the maternal microbiota.

A seminal study in 2004 using germ-free mice showed

that supplementation with probiotics of *bifidobacterium* and *lactobacillus* reduced stress and anxiety symptoms.[7] In another experiment germ-free mice received microbiota from obese mice and became obese.[8] When they received microbiota from lean mice, they became lean.

Gut bacteria can affect foetuses as well. For example, stress in a mother modifies her microbiota, which has been shown to increase anxiety levels in infants.[9,10]

The role of exercise in microbiota composition

The microbiota of exercising women has more *bifidobacteria* and *lactobacillus* compared to sedentary women.[11] These differences are independent of diet. They also have less of the inflammation-causing bacteria *staphylococcus*, *enterobacter* and *Escherichia coli* (*E. coli*).

It has been widely shown that a high-fat diet and sedentary lifestyle change the gut microbiota to promote low-grade inflammation in the tissues that can cause metabolic disorders and certain cancers. Initiating exercise before and during pregnancy protects the foetus from this inflammatory response, as exercise has been shown to change the composition of the microbiota.

This anti-inflammatory response due to physical activity protects the foetus from being rejected due to placental inflammation, particularly during the early phase of placental growth. It also improves placental functioning and increases nutrient delivery to the foetus. Rats with GDM showed a marked change in their gut microbiota when exercised, improving glucose tolerance in the offspring as well as the mother.

In another study a particular combination of microbiota showed improved endurance capacity.[12] Thus, it seems that healthy microbiota induce behaviours that promote physical activity. So this is a virtuous cycle of good bacteria influencing physical activity and exercise itself improving the microbiome.

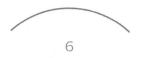

6

Preparing for the physicality of birth

In the 1600s François Mauriceau published an influential work on pregnancy and childbirth that popularised recumbent (lying down) birth positions, breaking thousands of years of traditional birth stool use.[1] Birth stools were used by midwives as far back as the 2nd century AD in Rome. Upright positions for birth were instinctively prized by women who understood how to make birth easier. These practises were also in line with their lifestyles, which included deep squatting and slow ambulatory work. Although he advocated recumbent positions, Mauriceau also promoted ambulation (gentle walking) during labour, suggesting that 'the woman being on her legs, causeth the inward orifice of her womb to dilate sooner than in bed; and her pains to be stronger and frequenter that her labour be nothing near so long.' He observed that moving more during labour and birth was beneficial and helped the body in its work of birthing the baby.

By the 20th century research suggested that recumbent and supine positions hinder blood flow and obstruct the pelvic passage more than upright positions, causing maternal and foetal distress.[2] Some studies have reported 35% less pain in the front and 50% less back pain in the back in upright positions compared to recumbent. This started a slow but definitive movement back towards being upright for birth.

Extensive research shows that there is no particular upright maternal position that is more or less favourable during labour, or that decreases the duration of labour. A recent systematic review and meta-analysis showed that hands and knees, side-lying or forward bends (creating a c curve in the spine) and being supported by walls or partners, are no better than other upright positions.[3] This makes sense, as we all have different anatomical and positional needs depending on the subtle uniqueness of our body's design, our baby's position relative to our pelvis, our habitual movements and mind-muscle links that we have created over an entire lifetime. The positions we assume at birth are what we feel most drawn to. There are some universal positions that suit most women, but if they are not for you, then you can do what your body and baby need without feeling that you are somehow compromising optimal positioning. The more you trust your body, the more natural the position will feel and will assist you and your labour. The trick is to stay mobile if you can, move a bit (ambulate), and let your body and baby move you without allowing your mind, which may be trapped in social norms and cultural restrictions, to get too involved. Simply, stay upright if you can.

How does being physically active help with birth?

Upright birth positions favour the use of gravity, which increases cervical pressure and thus uterine contraction intensity. This may lead to comparatively faster dilation. However, it has also been shown to increase fatigue. Fatigue in muscular activity manifests itself through reduced pH (the muscle cells becomes acidic) with a build-up of lactic acid and other by-products of energy expenditure.

When you train for a race or a sporting event, training the muscles and blood to sustain higher levels of acidity before they become fatigued is important. Athletes slowly increase the threshold at which they can continue to exercise. This physiological point is probably just as important to consider when thinking of birth preparation. Most birth preparation classes talk about positional and comfort-based techniques without paying much attention to the endurance and strength needed to birth a baby.

The physicality of birth has been left up to women to discover, while there has been so much talk about birth preparation that involves specific positions or techniques. In reality, these techniques and positions can only be employed if you can physically muster the energy, endurance and strength to use them. And that level of endurance doesn't come overnight. It requires physical strength that needs building up over time through physical activity.

During my first birth, I had a plan. I wanted to stay upright, I wanted to squat and birth my baby and I knew I wouldn't want to lie in bed. I had read all the reasons for staying upright and it all made sense. However, my birth was rather different to what I imagined. I was in labour for four days on and off. By the time it came to push the baby out, I was exhausted and simply didn't care about the position or anything. The birth wasn't the most empowering to be honest and I was so tired for weeks on end.

What I realised was in my second pregnancy I was a lot more active; I had a toddler to run around with,

I had taken up Zumba and started going to the gym. I don't think I did any preparation for birth as I didn't have any time. I was just generally healthier, and I am sure it played a part in me recovering more quickly. Lorna

Being upright throughout labour requires energy, endurance capacity and strength. Fatigue in labour is cumulative and intensifies as labour progresses. How can you possibly use positions like deep squats that involve most of the large muscles of the lower body and thus demand energy during the second stage, if the first stage has sapped most of your endurance? Repeated muscular contractions of the uterus and the surrounding larger muscles of the abdomen and hips all require energy and endurance. No wonder women need pain relief! An athlete in the middle of a race would be on his/her back asking for pain relief if they had not trained correctly.

Studies comparing the maternal cardiovascular system during labour to trained athletes show that the process of childbirth is not dissimilar to a long-distance race.[3] There are adaptations throughout your pregnancy that become important during birth, but nevertheless birth is one of the most physiologically, physically and psychologically demanding events of our lives.

The biggest demands during birth are placed on your cardiac system, followed by your muscular and endocrine systems. The demands are intense not just because of their similarity to moderate to high-intensity exercise, but also because of the duration of labour compared to sporting activities. Labour can take place over days, so the body requires physical adaptations that will delay fatigue for as long as possible and also make postnatal recovery quicker.

Cardiac output (a measure of circulating blood pumped

by the heart every min) dramatically increases during labour to levels seen in moderate to high-intensity physical training by non-pregnant people. The resting cardiac output for a non-pregnant person is around 5–6l/min. By eight weeks of pregnancy this can increase by 20%, peaking at about 7l/min around 24–28 weeks and staying that high for the rest of the pregnancy. This is partly due to increased blood supply demands that deliver oxygen and nutrients to your baby, but also to prepare your body for sustaining the physicality of labour.

In the first phase of labour, when heart rate increases to around 88 ± 10bpm (close to 100bpm during contractions), cardiac output can be as high as 10l/min. In comparison, cardiac output during low to moderate-intensity exercise can be around 9.4 to 17.5l/min. Most people would train at this intensity for a few hours at the most. Labour can last much longer.

The increase in muscular contractions during the second stage puts additional strain on both the muscular and the cardiovascular systems. Your heart rate can reach 90% of your maximal capacity. A study by Söchnchen in 2011 reported heart rate increases up to 172–188bpm.[4] Women who were less fit were much closer to their maximal heart rates than their fitter counterparts. These heart rate values correspond to people doing moderate to heavy exercise when not pregnant.

The lower your capacity to sustain high heart rates, the lower your cardiac output will be. This has serious consequences for oxygen and nutrient delivery to your contracting muscles. Lower oxygen makes the muscles accumulate more lactate, making them acidic. This means that muscular contractions have to slow down in order for the lactate to clear, potentially lengthening labour.

The capacity of your body to sustain higher levels of cardiac and muscular activities can be increased via long-term training and practice. Our bodies slowly learn to contract muscles in higher acidic environments, become better at clearing the accumulated lactate and do this with lower heart rates increases. This keeps fatigue at bay for longer.

Fatigue of labour is similar to fatigue of exercise, except it has the added element of mental fatigue, which plays a huge role in increasing the subjective feeling of fatigue. Most women respond to this fatigue by requesting pain relief, but that simply reduces the *perception* of fatigue, which might change behaviour to the point that mental fatigue can be managed. However, the reality of physical strain and the fatigue our bodies have to go through does not change. The only way this can be managed is by training our bodies to sustain higher levels of physical stress, and recover more quickly as a result of that training.

The fatigue of labour

During labour fatigue can develop physiologically, psychologically, because of certain situational factors, or a combination of these.

Physiological factors

1. ***Parity (number of pregnancies)***
   There is no statistical evidence that parity has an impact on labour pain, perception of pain or even pain-related behaviours. However, there are numerous anecdotal reports suggesting that if you have not given birth before your anxiety about the birth process can impact your pain perception and behaviour, influencing your energy levels.

2. *Uterine contractility*

    The more intense your contractions are, the more likely you will feel or be fatigued due to the high levels of energy needed. If you cannot sustain these intense contractions due to muscular fatigue (low oxygen, high lactic acid build-up), your labour may be lengthened.

3. *Sleep patterns*

    If you have had disturbed or reduced sleep in the last weeks of your pregnancy then this affects your energy levels and you may tire more quickly.

4. *Nutrition*

    Your blood sugar regulation determines your ability to maintain sustained physical efforts. Your haemoglobin levels maintain your oxygen supply.

5. *Exercise conditioning*

    Clapp in the 1980s, Pugh in the 1990s and latterly Lee in the 2000s have shown that women who stay active before and during their pregnancy report less fatigue than women who lead more sedentary lives. They have also reported that women with higher BMI show higher levels of fatigue during labour and longer recovery times. However, if the women with high BMI had stayed active throughout their pregnancies, they experienced lower levels of fatigue compared to those who didn't.

Psychological factors

1. Pain and the perception of pain have a huge impact on labour fatigue. Women with a history of menstrual pain, abortion, who expect less pain or who have unsupportive birth partners tend to perceive pain as more intense than others. The perception of pain or the inability to manage pain also causes hyperventilation, which increases acidity in the muscles and further reduces oxygen transfer to the

uterus at a time when oxygen needs are high. This classic negative oxygen delivery loop leads to earlier physiological fatigue.

2. Anxiety and fear of birth cause pain thresholds to decrease by increasing cortisol production, which enhances sympathetic nervous activity. High sympathetic nervous activity leads to adrenal stimulation, which consumes more energy, and a respiratory-cardiovascular environment (hyperventilation and decreased oxygen consumption) that prevents the judicious conservation of energy, leading to fatigue.

Researchers have found that even when women rate pain the same, their behaviour towards it depends on many factors such as cultural norms, ethnic and socio-economic backgrounds and preparedness for birth.[5] And although many women report labour pain as severe, they don't always view it as negative pain. Research also shows that women who experience painless or relatively painless labours do not seem to display any unique characteristics of pain management.

Situational factors

1. Pain medication decreases the perception of pain by reducing wakefulness, but since the physiological stimulation of muscles in labour is unaffected it can increase fatigue during and after labour. Once the medication wears off recovery from labour fatigue can be longer for women who have had pain relief compared to women who did not.

2. Occupational strain, anxiety and stress stimulate the sympathetic nervous system, releasing cortisol and increasing fatigue. By looking at these three aspects we

can see how regular, small amounts of physical activity before and during labour enhance the body's capacity to withstand muscular contraction and high energy demands for long periods. Regular physical activity also relieves stress and anxiety, and teaches your body and mind to manage the negative flow of energy-depleting stress hormones. This can also reduce the need for pain medication.

Mental resilience

The physical fatigue of birth is compounded by its deep connection with mental and emotional fatigue. No other competitive race or physical pursuit comes close to testing our mental and emotional resilience like birthing a new baby. All the elements of birthing a baby are fraught with risks and informed decisions. These decisions can be a great emotional and mental burden, as they may have far-reaching consequences for mother, baby, family and our society as a whole.

Mental health in pregnancy (and even pre-pregnancy) can play a big role at birth. Fears we may have held while pregnant or even before can manifest themselves as physical barriers at birth. Most of us do not get an opportunity to explore these barriers before birth. This means our stress and anxiety systems fire up and activate our sympathetic nervous system, impacting energy levels and causing fatigue.

When we feel emotionally drained our brain monoamine (serotonin, dopamine and nor-epinephrine) levels fall, we feel lethargic and tired and less capable of coping with the situation at hand. Like physical conditioning, regular exercise has been shown to improve our capacity to withstand mental pressures, thus dampening the impact of stress and anxiety.

Regular exercise also activates the monoamine system and increases the brain's capacity to withstand stress, feel less stressed at similar stress levels than before exercise training and, above all, improve recovery from stressful situations through becoming more resilient to stress over time. This long-term effect on stress and anxiety can be harnessed by keeping up your physical activity levels before and during pregnancy.

Exercise and oxytocin at birth

Labour is one of nature's paradoxes: the pain can be excruciating and yet amazingly positive. From an evolutionary perspective this may seem strange. Why would nature make childbirth so painful? Perhaps the pain involved in childbirth means the mother prizes the end result, encouraging her to take care of her baby.

The role of oxytocin in mothering activities is well established. However, new research is revealing the role of oxytocin in exercise psychobiology. Studies have shown that rhythmic cardiovascular activity increases oxytocin levels.[6] From a mechanistic perspective oxytocin has great advantages for the exercising individual, as it does for the birthing mother. Oxytocin acts as an analgesic and is involved in memory formation and recall. People who exercise for around 60 minutes show inflammatory markers in their blood (as exercise is a type of stress), but managing inflammatory markers helps create a pathway for your body to become more resilient. If oxytocin can reduce pain through its analgesic properties, then surely it makes sense that a body experiencing inflammation (and thus pain) will employ the oxytocin system to manage the pain. Thus, regular exercise improves our oxytocin system and regulation of pain and inflammation, which can be valuable during labour.

Even more interestingly, oxytocin's role in the memory of pain has parallels with exercise training. When pain is perceived as 'positive', such as during a marathon or labour, oxytocin has the ability to dampen the memory of its intensity. So, just like birthing women, people who exercise tend to perceive their pain as less intense than other kinds of pain such as surgery or dental procedures. This underestimation of pain and its memory takes place *during* the event rather than after. When circulating levels of oxytocin are high during exercise or labour, the memory records pain as of lower intensity. We need high levels of oxytocin for the pain to be remembered as lower intensity pain. People who exercise regularly display this as higher pain thresholds and an ability to tolerate situations of pain better than people who have not previously experienced the positive effects of oxytocin on the memory of pain.

Oxytocin also reduces fear and increases empathy by reducing activity in the parts of the brain where fear is felt. This is one of the reasons why, when we exercise, we feel good, confident and more social. The practice of feeling good and confident can then be taken into the labour room, where your labour will recreate that feeling you get from exercise and amplify the effects of oxytocin that you have experienced through a lifestyle that incorporates physical activity.

The rise in oxytocin helps in a couple of other metabolic events, such as maintaining fluid balance and regulating energy expenditure. High levels of oxytocin help us use fat as an energy source, sparing carbohydrates and protein to preserve lean tissue and preserving sugars for foetal supply during labour.

Women giving birth today have more 'managed' births than women in the past, for reasons including scientific knowledge and a culture of medicalisation of birth. As more women around the world experience these managed births, we are likely to lose our collective memory of the physicality of labour, the mental and emotional resilience needed, and what it may mean to 'dig deep' and find the strength we possess to birth our babies. I truly believe that physical fitness through prioritising physical activity allows us to approach birth ready to respond to pain and fatigue, which may make us anxious and fearful, from a starting point of strength and endurance.

Exercise and birth outcomes

Does exercise influence length of labour, type of birth; induction rates and instrumental delivery? Are fitter women really less likely to ask for pain relief? Are women who exercise at risk of preterm births?

In 2019 Maggi Davenport and her colleagues in Canada conducted a comprehensive analysis of the impact of exercise on birth outcomes, using data collated from 113 studies which amounted to 52,858 women.[7] They concluded:

> *Prenatal exercise was not associated with preterm/ prelabour rupture of membranes, caesarean section, induction of labour, length of labour, vaginal tears, fatigue, injury, musculoskeletal trauma, maternal harms or diastasis recti.*
>
> *Results from meta-regression did not identify a dose-response relationship between frequency, intensity, duration or volume of exercise and labour and delivery outcomes.*

Let's look at each variable further.

Does exercise influence the duration of labour?

Over the years various studies have tried to answer this question. However, the data does not provide a clear consensus. A large systematic review in 2014 looking at 855 exercising women who did some strength-based and aerobic exercise throughout their pregnancies found no impact of exercise on duration of labour.[8] In another study exercise in water for about 50 minutes had no significant impact on labour times, but women in the study requested significantly less pain relief.[9]

However, a smaller (140 women) Brazilian study in 2019 showed a 150-minute reduction in labour time in women who clocked up 60 minutes of exercise in the second and third trimesters.[10] There is also evidence that women who put on more weight during their pregnancies spend less time in labour if they stayed active (13.4hrs) compared to women who did not (19.2hrs).

There is growing evidence that the first stage of labour (cervix dilation of 4 to 10cm) is shorter in women who have been active through their pregnancies. In 2009 Kristin Kardel and colleagues quantified the fitness levels of women and correlated them with labour times. They found that women who had higher capacity to take up oxygen (one of the adaptations of regular physical activity) had shorter first stages. For every 0.1l/min more of oxygen uptake capacity, they saw a corresponding 30-minute reduction in labour time in first-time mothers.[11]

The second stage (from complete dilation to birth) requires muscular strength. Thus, pelvic floor-strengthening exercises have traditionally been considered beneficial. However, anecdotal evidence, particularly from the horse-riding community, suggests that a strong pelvic floor may causes the perineum not to yield during labour, making labour longer and resulting in corresponding perineal damage that negates any benefits of pelvic floor-strengthening exercises. Conversely, some evidence suggests that a strong pelvic floor may help the baby rotate and even reduce the incidence of instrumental delivery.

Leticia Dias and her colleagues in Brazil wanted to see if preterm labour in low-income Brazilian women could be influenced via pelvic floor-strengthening exercises.[12] They found no significant differences in the second stage of labour among women who exercised their pelvic floor specifically and those who didn't. In fact, another large compendium of studies looked at pelvic floor training and labour outcomes in 268 women and found no significant difference in pelvic floor strength and length of labour.[13] However, despite the lack of evidence on length of labour, it has been noted that a stronger pelvic floor leads to fewer 'pushes' in the second stage of labour. This demonstrates that a strong pelvic floor, despite not shortening the length of the second stage, does not obstruct labour. A strong pelvic floor will also help prevent urinary incontinence both antenatally and postnatally.

Does physical activity impact the type of birth?

Caesarean section

One of the biggest data sets (almost 93,000 women) comes from the Danish National Birth Cohort study (DNBC),[14] which reports that women who stayed physically active throughout their pregnancies had a lower chance of c-section births compared to women who did not (6% compared to 30%). Foetal stress, such as meconium, heart rate pattern and low Apgar scores were also reduced in exercising women. This is echoed by another large-scale analysis from Norway.[15]

Silveira and colleagues in 2012 split 66 women into two groups: a control group (who didn't do any specific exercise) and an exercise group (who exercised at moderate intensities in the second and third trimesters).[16] Vaginal births in the exercise group were 68% compared to 32% in the sedentary group. C-sections were up to 62% in the control group compared to 9% in the exercising group. Other studies have also shown a strong correlation between physically active women and increased incidence of vaginal birth.

Some 466 women were studied as part of the Growing up in Wales study, and the authors found that women who reported lower physical activity were more likely to have an instrumental delivery (including forceps, ventouse and elective and emergency caesarean) compared to mothers with higher activity levels.[17] Mothers with higher BMI (25+) were more likely to require induction, have a big baby and have a longer hospital stay after birth.

Instrumental births

Physically active women tend to have lower rates of instrumental births, with data from over 400 women in one study showing that instrumental birth rates in women who had reported high levels of physical activity were half (12.7%) compared to those who reported low activity (26%).[18] However, we must be cautious when interpreting the data, because vaginal birth rates are dependent on many other factors too. There are other studies showing no influence of exercise on the type of birth. It is difficult to isolate the effects of physical activity in the research.

Are women who have been active less likely to request pain relief?

As we have seen, pain and the perception of pain can be modulated by your ability to exercise. Exercise is a perfect stress-inducing activity to enable the body to adapt to future physical stress. It has been shown that people who exercise can withstand a wide variety of stress patterns. This involves their cardiovascular, respiratory, digestive, immune and lymphatic systems. Thus, the stress of labour can be better modulated by women who have adapted to physical activity.

The hormonal cocktail that reduces the perception of pain during exercise is also responsible for a similar effect during labour. In 2005 Hartman and his colleagues asked 50 women in labour to exercise for 20 minutes on a cycle ergometer.[19] They measured beta-endorphins at rest and after exercise. Endorphin levels after exercise were significantly higher compared to rest and 84% of the women rated their contractions as less painful. A similar earlier study of 36 women who exercised throughout their pregnancies found that these women had higher circulating endorphins than the women who didn't stay active during pregnancy.

However, pain is also correlated to pelvic size and orientation, the relationship of the baby's position to the pelvis and augmentation of contractions. Women who stay mobile tend to move in instinctive ways that allow for better foetal positioning than sedentary women, thus reducing the likelihood of pain related to foetal orientation during labour. The use of birthing balls and equipment otherwise used for exercise classes have shown to help in pain management and reduced use of analgesia.

Do women who keep active have reduced induction rates?

Induction of labour is a complex set of decisions based on various factors including maternal medical conditions and foetal health. It has been extremely hard for research to isolate the impact of physical activity on induction rates. Women with higher gestational weight gain, GDM and greater than 30 BMI have higher incidences of induction of labour.[20] All these conditions are improved when women engage in regular physical activity. So it is reasonable to believe that being more active can play in big role in decreasing rates of induction.

Are women who exercise at risk of preterm birth?

Preterm birth (before 37 weeks) is a major determinant of infant mortality (death) and morbidity (illness). Thus, if there are lifestyle factors that can influence preterm birth, such as physical activity, it is important that we know about them.

The data on preterm birth and physical activity differs depending on the *nature* of physical activity. Leisure activity, such as an exercise session, has a very different impact to occupational (work) physical activity.

Leisure activity

Most previous studies have found no link between leisure activity and preterm births. If anything, studies indicate that physical activity has a negative impact on preterm delivery. In 2017 researchers in Guangdong, China, investigated 849 pregnant women delivering preterm babies (PTB) and 1,306 delivering full-term babies in a case-control study.[21] They found that exercise frequency and duration were both negatively associated with preterm birth. In other words, exercise seems to reduce the risk of preterm birth. Placental weight (increased blood vessels in the placentas of exercising women) seems to be a major causal factor in this reduced risk.

A prospective study of 1,699 women in 2002 showed that even vigorous activity did not increase the risk of preterm birth.[22]

Occupational activity

Data spanning 20 years from 1987 to 2007 shows that prolonged standing for more than six hours increases risk of preterm birth. The standing posture encourages the uterus to relax, decreasing venous blood flow to the heart, which in turn increases foetal heart rate causing foetal distress. Some studies suggest that there is a link between certain activities such as stair climbing ≥10 times or walking for four or more hours per day and preterm birth. This data has been collected from women with low socio-economic status, which means that a lot of these activities might not be voluntary, and they may be done when the women are tired, increasing the risk of triggering contractions. This is corroborated by studies that show that the risk of preterm delivery is highest in women who stand for prolonged periods in their jobs compared to women who move a lot in their work.[23] Lifting heavy weights of more than 12kg 50 or more times a week has also been shown to increase the risk of preterm births. Women who have to continue physical activity despite feeling tired are at highest risk of preterm delivery.

Occupational physical stress, combined with the mental stress and pressures of a work environment, can come together to substantially increase the risk of preterm birth. If this affects you, raise it with your employer and consider getting external professional help to support you if necessary.

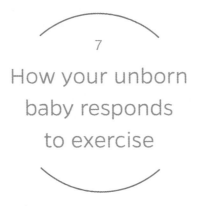

7

How your unborn baby responds to exercise

Growing your baby demands extra oxygen and nutrient uptake and better core temperature regulation and more efficient waste removal by the kidneys, among other things. So does exercise. Thus, it has been seen as reasonable to think that exercise, although beneficial to you, may not be of great benefit to your growing baby, as the two sets of needs will be in competition. In our culture we tend to consider the mother a vessel for carrying a baby, so we may even view women who exercise during pregnancy as selfish and not concerned about the impact on their babies. Until the mid-1990s the literature on exercise in pregnancy was peppered with statements about 'a lack of empirical evidence of exercise impacts on the baby' and exercise recommendations were considered 'controversial'. Papers referred to the intuitive understanding that exercise would divert blood flow from the growing foetus, impacting nutrient and oxygen delivery.

However, current research is challenging these assumptions and showing that we have underestimated the body's capacity for adaptation. During exercise there are some adaptations that require the foetal and placental systems to cope with a higher level of physiological stress. The response to this stress helps your baby adapt to survive challenging situations both in the womb and outside.

Normal growth curve of the foetus

If we look at the normal growth curve of a foetus, the growth pattern broadly looks like this:

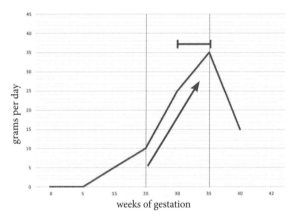

Indicative normal growth curve of a foetus.

We can see that the greatest rate of growth is from 20-32 weeks (arrow) and the greatest overall weight gain happens in from 30–35 weeks of gestation (marker at top of graph). Maternal adaptations to exercise, particularly in relation to the needs of the growing foetus for oxygen and nutrients, thus become challenging from 20 weeks onwards. You will put on a third of your pregnancy weight (~4.5kg) in the first 20 weeks, and two-thirds (~9 kg) in the second 20 weeks.

Oxygen delivery to the foetus

Exercising while pregnant has a beneficial physiological impact on foetal heart rate, cardiovascular systems and the general growth of your baby. The way in which the oxygen and nutrient delivery needs of your baby are met, while your blood flow is diverted to your exercising muscles, creates unique adaptations in your placenta and the foetal circulation.

A high demand for oxygen is complimented by a 10-fold increase in blood flow to the uterus from the beginning of your pregnancy till the end. Blood flow to the uterus is about 50ml/min in the first trimester, rising to more than 500ml/min by the third trimester. Your cardiac output (the total amount of blood your heart pumps in one minute) increases by 20% to accommodate this increase in blood flow. The major factors that determine oxygen delivery to your foetus are your cardiac output and your blood's ability to carry haemoglobin into the foetal circulation.

As your blood is directed away from your uterus during exercise, the transfer of nutrients (perfusion rate) is maintained. Within 5 minutes of starting exercise (cycling at low to medium intensity), the haemoglobin in your blood will start to increase and this increases oxygen delivery to the foetal-placental unit despite reduced blood flow. If you exercise regularly the foetal blood will contain higher amounts of red blood cells and the haemoglobin in them develops a higher affinity for oxygen. This allows your baby to withstand exercise-induced diversion of blood flow without compromising oxygen and nutrient delivery.

In one study, when women at 30–31 weeks of pregnancy performed a treadmill exercise at a rather high intensity (87–92% MHR), placental blood resistance decreased, allowing for more oxygen transfer to take place in the placenta.[1] Also, foetal heart rate increased by about 10bpm to compensate for the decrease in maternal blood flow to the placenta. When the foetal system detects a decrease in oxygen levels, it can activate vaso-active substances that decrease resistance in the arteries.

Despite needing a lot of oxygen, foetal arteries are not capable of carrying a lot of oxygen. Foetal arteries are 55–82% saturated with oxygen compared to the mother's oxygen saturation levels of around 97%, and no less than 95% during exercise. This is normal, as the baby generally survives and grows in a hypoxic (low oxygen) condition compared to his mother, despite his oxygen needs being almost twice that of adults. This means that when you exercise at a moderate to vigorous level you can still supply the right amount of oxygen to your baby, as your saturation will be no lower than 95% even then.

However, this is not true when other conditions are present, such as maternal smoking (carboxyhaemoglobinemia), sickle cell diseases (haemoglobinopathies) and maternal anaemia, all of which decrease oxygen delivery to the baby. If you suffer from any of these conditions seek appropriate guidance from both your doctor and a suitably qualified exercise professional.

Adaptations to the placenta

There are many adaptations to the placenta when you exercise during pregnancy, which protect your baby from a lack of oxygen or nutrients. For example, a 2000 study by James Clapp showed that when women exercised at a moderate intensity from about 8–9 weeks of gestation until birth, their placentas were significantly different from those of women who did not (the control group).[2] Exercise increased foetal-placental growth rate and placental growth was higher at ~20 weeks of gestation. The exercising women also had higher functional volume to their placenta and their babies were slightly bigger (not large for gestational age, but greater lean mass than the non-exercising women).

Clapp hypothesised that intermittent hypoxia (reduced oxygen delivery to the foetus) during exercise in early pregnancy coincided with the time when the placenta develops. Due to the exercise-induced low oxygen environment, the placental vascularity (blood vessels) compensated by making more (angiogenesis) and thicker blood vessels. So your exercise habit can inform the development of your placenta, and if your exercise needs divert blood away from the placenta then a more vascular placenta will ensure this will not be detrimental to your baby.

A more vascular placenta not only protects against diverted blood flow during exercise, but also has other protective benefits. A large recent systematic study has shown that women who exercised at intensities over 70% MHR had lower rates of preterm delivery compared to women who were sedentary (39+4 weeks vs 39+3 weeks).[3]

Impact on foetal heart rate (FHR)

Foetal distress is generally measured by change in foetal heart rate. A decrease in foetal heart rate (bradycardia) is a sign of foetal distress. Not many unborn babies display bradycardia as a response to maternal exercise. There is growing evidence on a wide range of maternal exercise that shows that exercise and physical activity is well tolerated by the baby. A systematic review of 91 studies looking at reports from 4,641 women reported low levels of bradycardia that corrected within 2 minutes of the end of exercise.[4]

Some studies have reported a small increase in FHR of about 5–10bpm, which returns to normal as soon as exercise ends. It is possible that small decreases in uterine blood flow cause the baby to stimulate chemoreceptors, which in turn stimulates production of catecholamines, which increase FHR. However, these chemo receptors in the baby are not fully developed till the third trimester. So, it is possible that catecholamine increase comes from your system when you exercise. Research indicates that about 15% of maternal catecholamines transfuse into the placenta, which could increase FHR. Therefore, a general increase in FHR when you exercise is not necessarily a sign of foetal distress.

There is very little data on exercise at more than 90% of your maximal capacity. One study reported a 12% decrease in uterine blood pressure but low incidence of bradycardia (0–3% of the sample) and low tachycardia (fast or irregular heart rate) (3–7%) in the babies.[5]

We still don't know the impact on the baby of a mother who suffers from pre-eclampsia or cholestasis (bile flow issues due to pregnancy hormones). So these specific conditions need individualised exercise monitoring. Bradycardia in the baby has also been reported when mothers exercise in supine (on their backs) positions.

We have no clear evidence of long-term impact on the foetus with bradycardia or tachycardia, related or unrelated to exercise, and the FHR changes reported in these exercise studies showed no association with increased numbers of c-sections, or implications for birth weight.

Impact on infant birth weight

Will exercise influence your baby's birth weight? Despite decades of research we still don't know the answer. While some studies report a reduction in birth weight in women who exercise, others suggest that larger babies are born to women who exercise. One reason for this is the complexity of isolating the impact of physical activity on birth weight. Birth weight is influenced by many interconnected factors.

We do know that both small for gestational age (SGA) and large for gestational age (LGA) babies experience long-term health effects.[6-8] Most studies have correlated an increase in birth weight with maternal weight gain, so exercising women who tend to put on less weight during pregnancy compared to sedentary women might have smaller babies. Staying physically active throughout your pregnancy is protective against excessive weight gain during pregnancy.

Some of the largest data sets, such as the Danish National Birth Cohort (DNBC) study (92,671 women)[9] and the Norwegian Mother and Child (MoBa) study (61,098 women)[10] have reported that women who take moderate exercise (50–70% MHR, can maintain a conversation) have a 30% less chance of an LGA baby and no increase in risk of an SGA baby.

Some smaller studies (400–500 women) have reported a small increase in birth weight (approx 100g) in babies born to women who undertook moderate intensity exercise. Clapp reported that babies born to women who exercised were larger but had higher lean mass rather than increased fat deposits.[11] This might be a consequence of maternal placental adaptations to improve oxygen-carrying capacity and increase haemoglobin.

None of the studies that reported increases or decreases in birth weight in exercise trials contained clinically LGA or SGA babies. The reported weight differences were small deviations from the mean.

Impact of your baby's birth weight on their long-term health

Your baby will generally grow according to your body size, rather than your genetic potential. In the womb, your baby can gather information on maternal size, age at pregnancy and whether they are your first baby from the physiological environment, placenta size and perfusion of nutrients. The baby's genes then respond to this anticipated external environment in order to give them the best chance of survival.

Some perinatal events, such as energy intake (nutrition) and energy expenditure (exercise) appear to exert effects on the birth weight of the baby that are independent of other environmental risks or amplify environmental risks.

Both SGA and LGA babies have been studied, and the impact of birth weight on a child's life into adulthood shows that at both ends of the spectrum there are increased risks of developing metabolic diseases such as diabetes, cardiovascular diseases including hypertension, osteoporosis and certain cancers. If your baby is born SGA then his risk of hypertension, type-2 diabetes and adult metabolic syndrome increases.[7] However, a baby born LGA has a 2–3 times increased risk of childhood obesity and diabetes as well, particularly if she is a girl.

It is not birth weight *per se* that is the risk, however: it is the slow gathering of information from the maternal physiology, which leads to a different pattern of programming of the foetal organs during in utero growth, that has an impact in later life. Something about the growth pattern triggers changes in the baby's DNA that predispose them to higher risks of certain diseases.

If an unborn baby is subjected to low nutrition early in his gestational life and then nutrition improves in late gestation, it has been shown that this programmes their organs to 'grow' more than 'repair' in later life. Such epigenetic changes have major health implications in adulthood.

A poor intrauterine environment leads to decreased skeletal mass and increased fat mass in babies. This is a good adaptation for survival, as the baby is being programmed for a poor nutrient environment outside the womb, based on the lack of nutrients he receives in utero. However, in the modern world, when they are born into an environment of surplus energy (food) availability, this leads to obesity and insulin resistance. Maternal exercise seems to mitigate this risk, as it has been shown that babies born to exercising women have more lean tissue and less fat mass protecting them against future obesity and diabetes.

Maternal hyperglycaemia (high blood glucose) tends to increase insulin in babies (hyperinsulinemia) and predispose them to higher fat deposits. There is now a strong body of evidence that suggests that obese mothers have children that grow up with increased risk of becoming obese and/ or diabetic themselves.[12,13] But if women exercise at low to moderate levels, their children show a marked decrease in risk of metabolic diseases. Studies looking at physical activity in overweight and obese pregnant women have shown that even small amounts of activity throughout pregnancy can have marked impact on both the pregnancy itself and the epigenetic markers of the babies.

Even though we do not have a lot of mechanistic studies yet, epidemiological studies (data connecting population-based variables with associations) are hinting that increased risks of certain cancers and other health outcomes can be traced to the uterine environment. The little we do know about the mechanism for this suggests that these changes happen in a tissue-specific region rather than the whole body.

There also seem to be some sex-specific changes. Mothers pregnant with boys who exercise seem to pass on different changes to their sons than pregnant women carrying girls.

How will exercise during pregnancy impact your baby's life in the long term?

Life has evolved under relatively toxic conditions. Toxin stress has been a factor in the genetic evolution of our ancestors. Environments of low oxygen, high acidity, radiation and so on have led to favourable adaptations that serve us well today. Our ancestors' physical activity levels had fitness consequences for their survival. The generation of free radicals (cell-destroying oxygen molecules) led to favourable adaptations in the evolution of our antioxidant system, which today guards us well against environmental and other pollutants, even lengthening lifespan by protecting our body against premature cell death. These same free radicals (by-products of energy expenditure) are also produced during exercise. Is it then possible that one of the drivers for epigenetic changes in our children is the level of our physical activity before, during and after pregnancy?

It is important to note the concept of hormesis in understanding how toxins helped create a better genotype. Hormesis is a concept used by toxicologists to explain the bell curve nature of the impact of toxins on body systems. There are stressors (toxins) that are beneficial to human evolution and epigenetic changes at low levels, and show an increasing dose-response relationship, but only up to a certain point. A very high dose has negative impacts on the body and its ability to adapt.

You can see a possible hormesis effect in maternal exercise: too little seems to negatively impact the baby, as sedentary pregnancies can increase the baby's chances of metabolic diseases later in life. On the other hand, excessive exercise also seems to impact foetal wellbeing and birth weight. In one study[14] women who did high volume, high intensity exercise (more than 50% of their pre-conception maximum capacity) had babies that were smaller compared to women who either did less or low-intensity exercise. These smaller babies are also at increased risk of metabolic diseases. There is growing interest in researching maternal (and paternal, up to fertilisation of the egg) physical activity across the perinatal period as a developmental stressor for the later health and wellbeing of children.

Are our children more cognitively able if we exercise during pregnancy?

A quarter of a century ago, Clapp (1996)[15] demonstrated that children of women who exercised during pregnancy retained the benefits at five years of age. The most surprising outcome of this work was the effect on cognitive function. Clapp reported that general intelligence and specific oral language skills of children born to active mothers were significantly higher than in children born to those who were sedentary during pregnancy. These outcomes were irrespective of socio-economic status and marital stability of the parents and all the children lacked formal pre-school environments.

In 1999[16] the same authors studied newborn babies and found that five days after birth, children of exercising women performed better in two of the six evaluations of the Brazelton Scale. This measures a newborn baby's response to their new environment, relationship to their parents and their individuality. The data has also been replicated at 12 months in a 2014 Brazilian study.[17]

By 2018 there was emerging evidence[18] of this effect at a molecular level. Brain-derived neurotrophic factor (BDNF) is a protein important in cognitive function that also plays an important role in neuroplasticity. This protein has consistently been shown to be present at higher levels in children born to exercising mothers.

Current and future research

Exercise has been shown to impact epigenetic changes in mouse offspring from mice from pre-conception, fertilisation (both father and mother), in utero and postnatally via maternal milk. Oocytes (female eggs) and sperm, as well as pathways involved in fertilisation are all altered by exercise. After fertilisation the influence of maternal exercise becomes more important than the father's. Mothers' exercise continues to be of value postnatally with the effect of exercise adaptations on breastmilk.

Favourable epigenetic changes in offspring have now been studied across various tissues of the brain (neurogenesis), heart, skeletal muscle and endocrine function (hormonal regulation that can ward off lifestyle diseases). Recent studies[19,20] have shown that maternal exercise impacts on glucose tolerance in offspring, reducing the risk of mammary tumours and Alzheimer's, and leading to better heart rate control and cell functioning in mouse offspring.

These changes occur in two ways, through changes in the DNA (methylation) or non-genetic changes in the RNA (via specific proteins). Both these pathways are impacted by maternal exercise as they are by other environmental stresses. This is how we constantly change our relationship to nature and adapt to survive. These changes stay with the offspring over 2–3 generations at least and then continue to modify. Thus, maternal physical activity can counter hard-programmed genetic propensity to disease in our children.

By being physically active during pregnancy and

breastfeeding[21,22] we are effectively communicating with the cells of our baby, programming them for a lifetime of resilience to environmental insults and fluctuations in energy intake.

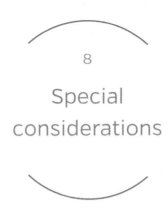

8

Special considerations

Although exercise in pregnancy and postnatally is generally beneficial for most women, there are certain situations which may affect the type of exercise you do or the duration, or may mean that you need to seek specific advice from healthcare professionals or qualified exercise professionals.

Physical considerations

Supine hypotensive syndrome (also known as Aortocaval Compression Syndromeor ACC)

From 20 weeks onwards, when the uterus is out of the pelvic cavity, the weight of the placenta, uterus, foetus and other tissues increases, so when you lie on your back the increased weight pressed into your back compresses a major vein (the superior vena cava) that sends deoxygenated blood back to the heart. It may also compress the major artery (aortacaval compression). This reduces the amount of blood available to pump around the body and the reduction in blood supply can cause mild discomfort in the short term (a couple of minutes) or even severe discomfort (nausea, light-headedness and fainting). However, vena cava compression and decreased blood flow can lead the sympathetic nervous system to compensate, which means you may not experience symptoms. If blood pressure drops by 15–30mm/Hg then you could experience pallor, dizziness, sweating, nausea and increases in heart rate, but in severe and prolonged conditions it may even lead to loss of consciousness.

The risk of adverse effects due to compression of the blood vessels increases if you have pre-existing blood pressure issues, especially pre-eclampsia, high BMI (more than 30), you are carrying multiple babies or have excessive amniotic fluid.[1] One of the bigger risks lies in reduced oxygen supply to the foetus (hypoxia), but this risk builds up over repeated compression of the vena cava, not a singular or isolated incidence. Some research suggests a reduction in uterine blood flow of up to 34% in supine positions.

Thus, it may seem that lying on the back during pregnancy (especially the second and third trimesters) should be avoided. However, despite the increase in certain risks, the research is clear that singular, short incidences do not increase risks to the mother or baby. Most research indicates increased risks in prolonged, static supine positions. Jeffreys in 2006[2] reported that exercise in supine positions is less vulnerable to these risks as decreases in blood flow in the supine position are two times lower when the lower extremities are kept mobile. So, lying on your back for short periods to exercise, especially when moving your legs, carries very little risk.

Here are some points to bear in mind if you choose to exercise in the supine position:

- If you have hypertension, pre-eclampsia or any heart condition avoid supine positions in the third trimester. If you have a history of small babies, intra-uterine growth restrictions (IUGR) or decreased foetal movements avoid supine exercise positions.
- In general, avoid lying supine when motionless and consider left lateral positions (side lying on the left) whenever possible, such as for sleep, medical examinations, labour and sex.

Deep Vein Thrombosis (DVT)

To prevent excessive blood loss during birth, pregnancy hormones increase the blood's capacity to clot (thrombosis). This is a protective mechanism, but other clinical risks may make deep vein thrombosis more likely. One way to reduce the chances of a thrombosis-related event during pregnancy is to move more. It has long been known that temporary immobilisation and physical inactivity are risk factors for increased thrombosis. Exercise, especially lower body movement, has been shown to decrease the incidence of deep vein thrombosis[3]. Studies have indicated that mild to moderate intensity exercise 2–3 times a week can significantly reduce the risks of deep vein thrombosis in women aged 15–44.

Nausea and vomiting

Nausea and vomiting (N&V) in early pregnancy affects 50–90% of women (hyperemesis gravidarum, severe N&V, affects 0.3–1% of all pregnant women)[4]. This can make exercising during the early stages of pregnancy extremely challenging. This can have a psychological impact if you are used to exercising before pregnancy. If you feel unwell, you should not ignore your discomfort in favour of the expected benefits of exercise.

Traditionally, increasing levels of HCG (human chorionic gonadotropin) have been thought to be associated with N&V in early pregnancy. However, not all women with high levels of HCG report symptoms of N&V, and not all women who report N&V have high levels of HCG. Emerging research is beginning to consider the role of psychological factors in developing N&V. A February 2020 study[5] of 1,682 women identified history of depression, plus high HCG levels at 12–14 weeks as significantly associated with N&V. Other studies looking at holistic measures of pregnancy wellbeing also report the association of psychological factors with developing N&V. Thus, although the current evidence on the management of N&V is poor, it is worth considering alternative ways of coping, such as cognitive behavioural therapy (CBT), mindfulness therapies and techniques of progressive muscular relaxation with stimulus control. So even if you cannot exercise, there are options that may help to manage your symptoms.

From a nutritional point of view, hydration is important. If you can find a tolerable drink, make an effort to keep drinking it. If the drink has a good balance of electrolytes, then that will also help maintain fluid balance, which can help manage the symptoms. Ginger and vitamin B6 (found in most cereals, eggs and vegetables or can be supplemented) may also help.

Muscular and anatomical conditions
Pelvic floor
Pelvic floor muscles are some of the deepest core muscles in our body, and they stabilise and assist in big core movements. New evidence[6] from anthropological data seems to suggest that the reasons we do not have a wider pelvis (as seen in other primates, making birth easier for them) are not entirely due to bipedalism (walking on our hind legs). It would have been possible to evolve with a wider pelvis to accommodate the

bigger brains our babies are born with, making childbirth easier and less dangerous, but this would have a massive impact on the pelvic floor strength needed to carry the unborn baby during pregnancy. It seems that our pelvis has evolved not to facilitate birth and walking, but to efficiently carry a baby to term over a long gestation period. The load on the pelvic floor grows exponentially as pregnancy progresses, so the pelvis has evolved to prevent prolapse and maintain the stability of the core.

This is an important consideration in the story of pelvic floor and its impact on pregnancy and childbirth. However, changes in hormones also cause the joints in the pelvis, and the cartilage and tendons that support the pelvic floor muscles, to become lax to facilitate childbirth. This laxity starts to create postural, strength and movement problems as pregnancy progresses, which can be a source of mild discomfort to extreme immobilising pain.

Compared to non-pregnant women there is a significant loss of strength of the pelvic floor muscles in pregnant women by the 36th week and after vaginal birth. Pregnancy makes the levator ani muscles stretch and thin, and conditions such as high BMI increase the risk of increased 'stretchiness' and decreased pelvic floor strength. Not only muscles, but also fascia and ligaments, are affected by hormonally mediated laxity. This also makes them less strong.

Does exercising the pelvic floor muscles improve their functionality?

The evidence is split on exercise and its impact on pelvic floor strength and functionality, for a few reasons. Firstly, there are many variations to the exercises, making it difficult to impose consistent regimes that can be studied and from which the results can be extrapolated into advice for practice. Secondly, the quality of the research design and the variations in the people studied, mean that simple conclusions are both naïve and perhaps misleading.

Classic 'Kegel' exercises have been recommended for decades. These are performed by isolating muscles (possibly levator ani) that are involved in urination. You are asked to imagine that you are trying to stop urinating mid-stream. Hold the contraction of these muscles for five seconds and release for five seconds and repeat.

The biggest barrier to the effectiveness of these exercises is that they require women to 'isolate' (be able to individually contract) muscles that are part of core muscular structures that work in tandem and support each other's function.

I had only been in the recovery ward for less than an hour, when a midwife came round for routine checks and asked me if I had started on my pelvic floor exercises yet? I could barely feel my body down there in the aftermath of birth and I couldn't even imagine trying to do any exercises. Just going to the toilet seemed like the biggest hurdle at the time. Jennifer

It is almost impossible for new starters to know whether they are truly isolating the required muscle, or whether some other synergistic muscle is performing most of the work. Isolating deep, core muscles is very hard to learn and do. So, it is not that Kegels do not work, it's just that most of us do not do them in textbook fashion. Most of us use our abdominal, thigh and buttock muscles, so we do not affect the strength of the pelvic floor.

In my experience as a former bodybuilder and student of yoga, practices that involve core muscle activation through controlled breath modulation, and holistic body movements that involve big muscle groups such as squatting, are more effective in maintaining and improving pelvic floor strength. In such exercises the whole pelvic floor has to function effectively with the core abdominal muscles, thighs, back and buttocks. This is what exercise scientists' term 'functional strength'. Instead of trying to isolate muscles and contract them, exercises to strengthen the pelvic floor have to mimic what it is designed to do. For example, squatting down or reaching up or twisting the torso are fabulous ways to engage the core and by default the pelvic floor, which has to engage to support the core. Moreover, these big movements build whole-body strength. When women are not asked to think about isolating singular or small groups of muscles and simply perform an activity such as a squat, they invariably contract the right muscles. This needs to be balanced with correct breath modulation too, because the core reacts to the thoracic cavity changing shape while breathing and this forms an important part of the movement.

Looking through the conflicting evidence on pelvic floor exercise regimes, it seems research supports this view. A recent Cochrane review[7] of almost 10,000 women from 38 different research studies from 20 countries shows that pelvic floor exercises done before urinary incontinence began had a positive effect in reducing the incidence of urinary incontinence during pregnancy and soon after childbirth. However, there was no evidence that this helped in the long-term postnatal period. However, women who already suffered with urinary incontinence saw very little impact on their condition or quality of life. The same was true of faecal incontinence, although there is less data.

Does pelvic floor exercise have an impact on labour duration or outcomes?

Most research on pelvic floor exercises concentrates on incontinence. However, arguments about a strong pelvic floor obstructing labour, or facilitating labour, are made in various publications. One study looked at differences between women who did pelvic floor exercises (similar to Kegels) and women who did not. Researchers were looking for differences in the second phase of labour and the incidence of instrumental birth. They found no difference in rates of caesarean section between women who did pelvic floor training and those who didn't. Pelvic floor training did not seem to impact either the second stage or other birth outcomes such as epidural rate, episiotomy rate or degree of perineal trauma. This was a secondary analysis of data collected for a study looking at urinary incontinence, and women who participated already had some degree of urinary incontinence. It supported findings from other studies in showing that training the pelvic floor muscles helps in the short-term management of urinary incontinence especially if started before the condition develops. However, the most interesting point is that pelvic floor exercises neither hinder nor help with childbirth itself.

Pelvis and lower back pain

50–75% of pregnant women are estimated to suffer from some sort of pelvic and back pain during pregnancy 25–40% of these women continue to have pain up to a year postnatally, and 1 in 10 women will still feel the impact of the pain over a decade later. The different types of pain can be categorised based on where they are felt and what kind of functionality they impact.

Lower back pain (LBP) starts around the lower thoracic (T10–12) discs and into the lumbar region (L1–5), sacrum and tailbone down to the gluteal fold (bottom part of the buttocks where the thighs start). If the pain is restricted to the pelvic area, where the hip bones join the sacrum and into the bottom of the buttocks, it is known as pelvic girdle

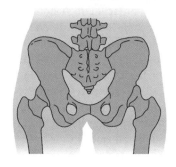

Site for pelvic girdle pain

pain (PGP). Some women have one type of pain or the other, whereas some suffer from both together, which is known as lumbo-pelvic pain (LPP).

Pain in the back and pelvis can cause significant disruption to sleep, work, social and sexual life. Ironically, this discomfort can put women off exercising. Three recent large-scale analyses of various small studies have revealed a clear picture of the role of exercise in the management of LPP during and after pregnancy.

The biggest is a 2018 analysis which informs part of the new Canadian exercise guidelines[9], which studied 52,297 women. It shows that exercising does not decrease the odds of *developing* LPP, either during or post-pregnancy. However, exercise is better than non-exercise in managing the pain and improving quality of life during pregnancy and the postnatal period.

Another analysis of 39,184 women from the Norwegian Mother and Child cohort (MoBa study)[10] showed that women who exercised 3–5 times a week had a 14% reduction in risk of developing PGP. High maternal BMI and increased maternal age (over 40) were both associated with higher risks of developing PGP.

A 2015 Cochrane review[11] of 5,121 women showed that land-based exercises significantly reduced pelvic pain, but manual therapies such as acupuncture, along with exercise, might be more effective. This is important to consider, as medication use can be restricted during pregnancy and breastfeeding.

How does exercise help in pain management?

The most important aspect of exercise is that it can maintain strength and flexibility of the muscles surrounding the lower back and pelvis, which improves load distribution on the spine and thus joint stabilisation and spinal alignment.

We still don't know which types of exercises best relieve LPP, or when is an appropriate time during pregnancy to start exercise specific to LPP. Movements that involve flexion (bending forward), extension (gentle back bends) side bends and rotation of the torso all seem to improve spinal alignment and joint stabilisation. These are actions that the pelvis and the lower back are involved in, and thus the functional strength from such movement improves the functional capacity of the pelvic musculature. Exercises that incorporate strength with flexibility have a greater impact than repetitive aerobic-type exercises.

There are many different types of stretching. Static stretching, where you hold the stretch, is the most effective form of stretching for LPP. It is important that stretches are held for no more than 30 seconds, and repeated no more than 2–4 times, as there seems to be no benefit beyond this range. These stretches may induce mild short-term discomfort, and stretching within the painful range (dull achy pain, rather than sharp shooting pain) is safe. Exercise consultants should feel confident in prescribing stretches that may be uncomfortable. Most GPs and midwives are not trained in exercise prescription and thus often do not feel confident in prescribing the right dose of exercise to make LPP pain manageable, so consult a specialist exercise professional if you need advice.

Symphysis Pubis Dysfunction (SPD)

The symphysis pubis is the small point in the front of the pelvis that brings together the two pelvic halves in the front of the body. Like all joints and ligaments it relaxes in pregnancy due to hormonal changes. In some cases, this can cause mobility issues and/or pain. Interestingly, the intensity of pain is not associated with the degree of movement or separation.

Factors such as heavy manual work, bad posture and lack of muscle strength in the core and the pelvic floor contribute to the condition. A previous history of difficult births, including shoulder dystocia, is a risk factor in subsequent pregnancies.

The pain associated with normal movements and activities can be severe for some women and affect their quality of life dramatically. Once the condition develops and the pain 'settles in', it becomes harder to tolerate exercise, resulting in a vicious

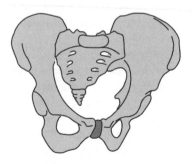

Symphysis Pubis shaded dark

cycle of deteriorating muscular strength and worsening pain.

If the pain is mild to moderate, carry on exercising. Research shows that exercise prior to and before the pain settles has a protective effect on the incidence and severity of SPD. Core stabilising and pelvic floor-strengthening exercises help stabilise the SPD-related compensations of postural alignment and movement. If the pain is severe, movements such as opening the thighs and walking can become very difficult. It is unlikely that hip-opening exercises make the condition worse, but they may increase short-term pain.

Generally, as this condition is both hormonal and due to the load exerted by pregnancy, it resolves itself after birth. However, if you experience continued pain, consider seeking a referral to an experienced physiotherapist.

Diastasis recti

The weight of your growing uterus sits predominantly in your abdominal cavity. With changes in your centre of gravity and the consequent reduction in core stability, muscles, connective tissue and fascia are compromised. Moreover, the hormonal thinning and stretching of these tissues leads to further loss of strength.

More than half of all pregnant women experience some form of reduction in core strength and functionality. By 22 weeks of pregnancy, when your uterus slowly comes out of your pelvic cavity to support your growing baby, you will start to feel the impact of these changes in your core abdominal area. The biggest muscle, the rectus abdominus, continues to be compromised in strength and functionality until the end of pregnancy, which means the effects last into the postnatal period.

When the muscle thins and starts to separate more than 2 to 2.7cm, it is known as diastasis of the rectus abdominus muscle (DRAM). DRAM impacts trunk movement, pelvic stability and postural alignment, which then impacts movement and increases risk to surrounding muscles that may have to compensate for the lack of core strength.

DRAM tends to resolve naturally after birth. C-section, carrying heavy loads with inappropriate techniques and some medications can affect natural recovery. After 8–12 weeks natural recovery plateaus, but even after that there is evidence to suggest that unless the separation is more than 4cm, intervention may not be necessary unless it impacts function. If you are concerned, it might be a good idea to refer yourself to a qualified professional who may be able to prescribe the correct exercise for your circumstances.

I was surprised to find that at my 6-week check the GP said that I had separation in my abdominal muscles and I must not do exercises for a while. I had a normal (sic) birth and I didn't feel like I was in any pain, so this diagnosis came out of the blue. I went home and did some research and decided I needed to talk to a physio about this rather than just not doing any exercise. The physio was very good at examining me thoroughly and then gave me a few exercises which were more about slow breathing than anything else and I did them every day. I am now 6 months postnatal and the separation has gone away. Claire

In the recent years, I have noted anxiety among pregnant and new mothers about DRAM. I think this is due to an increased awareness of the condition in mainstream and social media. I am keen to reassure you that most cases of DRAM resolve with normal life activities. You can help yourself by considering posture, alignment and using big muscle groups rather than inefficient ways of pulling and pushing. For example, use your back muscles to pull something rather than your small arm muscles.

What types of exercise may benefit recovery from DRAM?

Targeting the deeper transverse abdominal muscles (the ones that run diagonally across the torso) via a series of trunk rotation movements may be beneficial, as it strengthens the connective tissue and stimulates fascia growth and elasticity.

For improving the general integral strength of the core, breath-based thoracic movement exercises have been shown have maximum impact[12,13]. For example, as you exhale, slowly draw your belly button back into your spine. You can do this lying, sitting or standing. The way to gently progress is to increase exhalation time rather than force the belly button in. Keep the breath flowing and moving and pay attention to not holding the breath at any point in the cycle. This may seem simple, but this level of core activation will help natural recovery.

It may seem counterintuitive, but is important *not* to do crunches and abdominal flexion-based exercises, particularly those in which you 'pulse' at the midpoint of the crunch. These exercises cause more damage in the long run, lengthening the time to recovery and delaying muscle fitness.

Other exercises that may impact recovery times negatively are isometric contractions of the core such as planks. It's best to keep intense core activation exercise for 8–12 weeks after birth. This is to ensure that natural healing is not compromised. You can, however, gradually resume these activities over time.

In general, most research suggests that physical activity, especially before and in early pregnancy, is protective against pelvic and lower back pain. Continuing to move is generally a better idea than being sedentary. Mild pain when exercising is not harmful if it is monitored and managed by a qualified exercise professional. In the case of DRAM, SPD and to some extent even pelvic floor strength, the best strategy is to not embark on any specific exercise regimes soon after birth, as these issues tend to resolve naturally. However, if you continue to be affected by any of these conditions beyond 12 weeks after birth, seek individualised care rather than employing generic exercise regimes that may not be appropriate for your specific needs.

Physiological conditions
Gestational diabetes mellitus (GDM)

Diabetes UK estimates that about 16 in 100 women may develop GDM. There is mounting evidence that exercise pre-conception and during pregnancy is protective against developing GDM. This reduces the risk of type-2 diabetes in both mother and baby later in life. The evidence for exercise as part of a strategy to manage GDM is strong. In a recent systematic review and meta-analysis[14] of 1,875 women, those who were active before and during pregnancy significantly reduced their risk of developing gestational diabetes.

Another study[15] of over 900 pregnant women showed that those who were active a year before they got pregnant had a 66% reduced risk of developing gestational diabetes compared to the general population risk, and those who started exercising during pregnancy had a 33% reduced risk. The women who were active both before and during their pregnancy reduced their risk of developing GDM by 77%. If the pharmaceutical industry got such clear results about a drug treatment, they would be letting us know from every billboard possible.

However, current guidelines on exercise during pregnancy do not give adequate information about how to exercise to prevent or manage GDM. Conventional management strategies are still heavily biased towards diet and insulin-based interventions, with only vague exercise guidelines.

When I was diagnosed with gestational diabetes I was sent to a dietitian who gave me some good tips on modifying my diet. But she didn't talk about exercise or anything. I had been very poorly in my first trimester and had stopped most of my exercises and was still not doing much. I found it hard to restart and didn't have much motivation. But had I known how much exercise would have helped my diabetes and all the benefits it has for my baby, I think it would have been the motivation for me. From my experience, I can say that there was a lot of information on diet but not on exercise. Anon

During pregnancy, increased insulin insensitivity increases the risk of developing gestational diabetes. Exercise (particularly big muscular contractions) activates an enzyme called AMPK in the muscles, which can drive glucose into the exercising muscles without insulin. Activation of AMPK is one of the ways in which the diabetes drug Metformin manages blood glucose levels. Thus, if we engage in resistance exercise, we can mimic the action of Metformin.

Resistance exercise seems to have a strong protective effect on GDM incidence and management, and a combination of aerobic and resistance exercise at least three times a week at a moderate level (BORG intensity 12–14) is ideal. Resistance exercise three times a week for 30 minutes has been shown to reduce the chance of developing gestational diabetes and poor perinatal outcomes. A randomised control trial of 91 women conducting 35 minutes of moderate intensity exercise with 25 minutes of resistance exercise three times a week reduced risk for developing gestational diabetes by 27%. Studies looking at women with obesity who were undertaking moderate exercise have not demonstrated such large reduction in the chance of developing gestational diabetes, but other beneficial outcomes, such as a reduction in newborn body weight above

4kg, were significant outcomes of the exercise programme in these women.

While medication may be necessary for women whose blood glucose levels need to be managed, it is important to remember that exercise has shown no risk of adverse outcomes in pregnancy. Indeed, it should be the first line of strategy in prevention of GDM, for both better birth outcomes and long-term health benefits for mother and baby.

It is important to note that exercise may increase the risk of hypoglycaemia, which will affect women who may be on insulin therapy. Appropriate medical advice and support from qualified exercise professionals is of paramount importance for these women.

Pre-eclampsia

About 2–8% of women worldwide suffer from pre-eclampsia during pregnancy. Pre-eclampsia increases sympathetic nervous system activity, causing blood vessels in the placenta to reduce blood flow to the uterus, among other complications. Existing chronic hypertension, obesity, kidney dysfunction, increased maternal age and multiple pregnancies have all been identified as risk factors for developing pre-eclampsia. Getting pre-eclampsia also increases a woman's risk for later life hypertension, cardiovascular and renal disease and there is growing evidence of increased risk of dementia and Alzheimer's too.

Maternal anxiety levels have been shown to increase the risk of hypertension in pregnant women[16]. Regular physical activity helps lower anxiety and increase in systolic blood pressure, which may protect against pre-eclampsia. Physical activity also strengthens the cardiovascular system, improving the ability of the blood vessels to function, and increases production of neurotransmitters such as endorphins.

In addition, long-term exercise improves antioxidant and anti-inflammatory capacity. As exercise creates more inflammation and oxidation in cells due to increased energy expenditure, the long-term benefit of exercise is that the body adapts by increasing antioxidant and anti-inflammatory molecules. These specialist molecules also help maintain good placental function, reducing the risk of pre-eclampsia.

There have been a few studies showing a negative impact of exercise on pre-eclampsia risk. These studies have either been looking at high-intensity exercise, when there is a greater reduction in blood flow to the uterus than during moderate exercise, or women who had a higher risk of developing pre-eclampsia and were put on an exercise regime while they were pregnant. Looking at the research design reassures us that exercise does not increase the risk of pre-eclampsia in most cases.

Anaemia

Increased demand for iron for the growing baby, as well as for the blood and other tissues, sometimes creates an iron deficit during pregnancy. Iron deficiency anaemia (less than 11g/dl of iron in the blood) can lead to fatigue, decreased work performance and increased stress on the cardiovascular system. Iron deficiency can also lead to depressed immunity and poor tolerance of heavy blood loss during birth.

Research indicates there is no additional risk from exercise in developing anaemia. A Spanish study [17] in 2009 divided 160 pregnant women into two groups, a control and a group that exercised twice a week for 35–40 minutes. Researchers found that exercise did not reduce iron levels in pregnant women. However, heavy exercise leads to increased breakdown of cells and sweating, which can increase iron loss. Pro-inflammatory molecules such as cytokines, produced during heavy exercise, can also have a negative impact on iron transport.

Exercising when you have iron deficiency is not harmful, but fatigue and reduced oxygen transport due to low iron can make exercise and physical work harder. It is best if the iron deficiency is resolved through supplementation or other pharmacological means before embarking on an exercise regime. Rest and hydration are important when you take up exercise after being anaemic. Do not overexert yourself or tolerate light-headedness, and stop if you experience discomfort. Consult appropriate professionals for guidance if necessary.

Multiple pregnancies

In many ways multiple pregnancies are physically more demanding than carrying a single baby. Women tend gain on average 3.5kg more weight carrying twins, and there are some differences in the pattern of weight gain. Women with multiple babies tend to put on more at the start (water retention and tissue growth) and at the end of the pregnancy (baby weight) compared to women with single babies who put on most weight in mid-pregnancy. This may sometimes mean that exercise is adapted slightly for women pregnant with twins and multiple babies.

Remarkably, most women will not experience significant differences in their adaptations to pregnancy due to multiple babies. Most research indicates that cardiovascular adaptations such as cardiac output (the amount of blood pumped in a minute) do not differ significantly in multiple pregnancies. Some women may experience a faster heart rate. Even normal dietary intake is unchanged for most multiple pregnancies, as your body just becomes far more efficient in absorbing more nutrients.

However, despite the similar physiology of singleton and multiple pregnancies, the lived experience can be very different for some women. Increased uterus size can be a cause of more backaches, and pressure in the abdominal cavity can cause more issues with passing urine, constipation, varicose veins and oedema. Sometimes the physical discomfort of breathlessness can be exacerbated. Thus, exercise at intensities that allow normal conversations are likely to be more sustainable. Yoga, swimming and small frequent bouts of exercise can be better tolerated. You should certainly prioritise relaxation and release of tension to improve physical comfort.

Injury prevention and care in special situations
High-altitude exercise

Altitudes higher than 2,500 metres present unique problems for normal survival, and this is compounded by the physiological changes of pregnancy. When we include exercise things become very complicated and demand extra caution.

A few weeks of altitude living has been shown to change placental growth and function. People living and working at high altitudes have thicker, heavier and larger placentas to ensure oxygen delivery to the baby. There is more capillary density to increase the distribution of the oxygen through increased uterine blood flow, thus protecting the baby against hypoxia.

If you come from a culture that has generations of high-altitude living, you will benefit from long-term adaptations such as changes in the shape of your chest cavity to allow for deeper breathing. If not, your body will still make some quick adaptations within days, such as changing your breathing pattern. Although there are challenges and precautions are needed, pregnancy need not stop you from enjoying some high-altitude activities.

If you are going on a hiking or skiing holiday, your first consideration should be getting some rest at altitude. Make sure you take a few more days than you would ideally need.

This means you do not start exercising on the day you arrive and give yourself a few days to acclimatise.

Start at lower altitudes (1,800–2,000m) for 4–6 days if possible before ascending any higher. The more intense the activity, the lower the altitude should be. Also, avoid going to higher altitudes if you have compounding issues such as high blood pressure, severe anaemia or foetal growth issues due to a pre-existing heart or cardiovascular condition.

Diving

The risk of diving during pregnancy remains unclear, and ethical barriers to research mean that we may never fully understand it. Most of the current data we have on the physiological consequences of diving come from men and non-pregnant women. There is some evidence from pregnant women who chose to dive either because they were unaware of their pregnancies (early pregnancy), or were unaware of the risks involved.

The potential hazards of diving are oxygen toxicity and nitrogen gas bubbles getting embedded in joints and tissues. We do not know how foetal tissues respond to these bubbles. It has been suggested that diving at a depth of more than 60 feet might not be suitable during pregnancy. Retrospective evidence suggests that a one-off dive if you are not aware of being pregnant, provided decompression procedures are appropriately carried out, does not pose a high risk to either you or your baby, and abortion is not recommended. It is repeated exposure to over-saturated gas levels that could lead to potential issues with foetal growth and birth outcomes.

Professional athletic activities

In 1948 Francina Blankers-Koen won gold in 100m, 200m, 80m hurdles and 4 x 100m relay while she was three months pregnant. She may have trained for most of her events before she got pregnant, but she demonstrated that being pregnant was no barrier to high physical activity levels. Other athletes including Joan Benoit-Samuelson (1984 Olympics and 1987 Boston Marathon), Lorraine Moller, Paula Radcliffe and Kara Goucher have also demonstrated that with proper individualised care, normal low-risk pregnant women can train at elite levels while pregnant.

More and more women are participating in sporting events and we need clear guidelines that support physical activity at a high level during pregnancy and after birth. One of the barriers to achieving this is that the pool of professional athletes to study is too small to allow the data to be extrapolated more generally. However, growing numbers of studies are helping create a more robust picture of the upper safe limits in terms of exercise tolerance to maintain pregnancy and for foetal wellbeing. A study[18] looking at 26 professional athletes compared the raining regimes of the athletes with birth outcomes and found that endurance training was positively correlated to birth weight and strength straining was negatively correlated to foetal complications during pregnancy.

Most professional athletes train at a high level, with much of their training regime at high intensity, also called 'vigorous' exercise. 'Vigorous' is not well defined in the scientific literature and can range from 60–80% of maximal capacity. A study[19] of 45 low-risk pregnant women set out to identify the upper safe limit of exercise for this population. The researchers divided the women into three groups of 15: one group did no exercise (less than 20 minutes a day), one did mild-moderate exercise (around 20 minutes of exercise three days a week) and one did vigorous exercise (more than 20 minutes, more than four days a week). They tested each group, increasing effort until the participants gave up. In all groups the measures of foetal wellbeing were reassuring. Two participants had their heart rate exceed 90% of maximal capacity, but this did not affect foetal wellbeing. Another similar study found foetal wellbeing was reduced at intensities over 90% maximal capacity.

Thus, it seems from the current evidence that women who are already well trained can continue to train at a high intensity up to 90% of their maximal capacity. There seems to be some evidence of foetal distress (no data on long-term impact) above that threshold.

A study[20] by Kristin Kardel in 2005 aimed to identify whether *high-intensity* exercise could be replaced by *high-volume* exercise to maintain fitness levels in extremely well-trained women. Kardel studied pregnant athletes who had been training at a high level for at least 12–15 years. The women were asked to pick either a moderate training volume (90 minutes per session; 6 hours/week) or high training volume (150 minutes per session; 8.4 hours/week) from 17 weeks gestation to 12 weeks postnatal. She found that women on the high-volume programme did not lose their fitness levels at six weeks postnatal. This showed that high-volume training was well tolerated among previously well-trained women without loss of fitness. If you are an athlete these sorts of innovative changes to your training programme can help you modify and alter your training regimes under supervised guidance.

It is important that we find ways to support women who want to continue to train at high levels during and after their pregnancies. Research indicates that most professional athletes do not wish to end their careers due to being pregnant or becoming parents. Like most individuals, professional athletes find lack of time (especially childcare responsibilities) a great barrier to their training goals. In order to support professional athletes to train during and after pregnancy, we need to create policies and an environment that motivates, supports, and builds confidence.

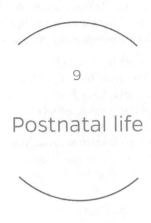

9

Postnatal life

The moment your baby arrives in the world is imprinted on you at the deepest level. Some of us experience unadulterated joy, pride and fulfilment. Some of us encounter bewilderment and a sense of overwhelm. We might even enter motherhood in a dark cloud of uncertainty and fear. Whichever path we're on, we proceed on this transformational journey in our own unique way.

In the early hours, days and weeks, as we adjust to our new identity, perhaps we feel a vague distance from that person who was pregnant and went into labour. On the other side we are floating in a world where the voices around us are familiar, our things are exactly how we left them, but our bodies and minds have altered irrevocably.

One of the first jolts of the present reality for me as a brand-new mum, was the experience of my phantom pregnant belly as I washed myself a few hours after the birth of my son. I recollect that out of body experience as I stood under the shower, water trickling down my body, that sense of acute newness to my physicality. Debbie

When we put on a bit of weight or lose a little bit, it's so subtle that we don't have to deal with or process dramatic change. But a postnatal body is an experience that is totally different, and that can come as a shock.

We suddenly feel the loss of our gorgeous massive belly, a loss so quick that at no other time in our lives do we experience such a vast contrast in our bodies. How can we deal with this alongside all the other challenges of mothering?

Let your breath do the talking

In the early days, when your body is responding slowly to its new role, there's a great opportunity to set up a practice of breath awareness that is the first step on the road towards more physically demanding exercise later.

The beauty of meditative, mindfulness practice is that it doesn't require you to choose yourself over your baby. It's an egalitarian practice of bringing your baby into your world, introducing your personal identity to your child and letting him get to know you as an individual and as a partner. *Just sit with your breath, notice it.* A great way of making this into a practice is to incorporate it into an activity that you do regularly, such as feeding your newborn. Every time you feed (breast or bottle), watch your baby and go internal and watch your response to your baby. How does your breath, the master communicator of your physiological environment, respond to your mothering task? Just watch and accept. Don't argue back, don't compare and certainly don't demand. If your attention drifts away, that's fine. Just bring it back whenever you realise you are miles away on a train of thought.

I still vividly remember the first few hours when we came to the recovery ward. It all felt a bit alien, I don't know how to describe it. It was noisy, bright and there was always some flurry of activity. There were visitors and midwives and trolleys that's all I remember. I used to sit there feeding my baby looking at it all and remember feeling a bit panicky. I didn't know why I felt that way. My partner tried to reassure me it was my birth hormones, but I knew that was not true. I wish I had some better coping strategies and these things are not talked about in antenatal classes. But from speaking to other mums, I know now that many felt overwhelmed with their environment, including the ones who had their babies at home. Susan

By creating this simple routine, you are making space for self-care and this will also help you manage your emotions and environment as a new mother. Over the coming weeks you can build on it to incorporate physical exercise. First, add straightening the spine to the breath awareness after a couple of weeks. Now you have the added advantage of a less sore back – back pain is often caused by slouching while you feed. Working on better maternal and postnatal posture is one of my starting points when I work to introduce physical exercise to new mothers in my professional capacity. I consider this to be a more immediate need than the pelvic floor exercises that are mostly recommended.

Giving attention to the birthing seat: pelvic floor

Now that we've begun to address mindfulness and posture, we can consider the specific aspects of our body that have a tough time while birthing our babies. Bring your daily practice to your pelvic health. Most current evidence suggests it is never too early to think about your pelvic floor musculature. Research[1,2] indicates that if you can start to consider your pelvic floor within 24 hours of birth, you should. This initiates early soft tissue repair and over the coming weeks and months more specific musculature and connective tissue healing can ensue.

However, if you feel too much pressure to do these specific exercises, don't worry. Even if you don't start pelvic floor exercises until a few weeks after birth, there is enough evidence to suggest you can make a good and full recovery over time[2,3]. Prioritise getting your mind comfortable with the idea of an exercise routine. This will make it easier to stick to in future.

Another reason why I advocate building a breath awareness practice before pelvic floor exercises is that many women hold their breath and contract their abdominal and gluteal muscles while doing pelvic floor exercises, which is counterproductive. If you can enjoy your breath, and the moment in which you can sit and observe it, *you are likely to naturally elongate your exhalation*. This is a by-product of stimulating more of your parasympathetic nervous system, which is exaggerated when you feel calm and at peace. *This elongated exhalation allows you to contract and 'lift' your pelvic floor up, rather than squeezing it in like a sponge.* The subtlety of this change in movement makes a world of a difference when it comes to reducing urinary incontinence (affecting 64% of new mums) and faecal incontinence (10% of us will suffer).[1]

But what about fitness?

Unlike our grandmothers and mothers, we live in an age where our bodies are a big part of our identity. Postnatally, we may feel lost. We who ran marathons, scaled large walls in climbing centres and did charity hill walking are used to our bodies working hard for us. We are not told that birth is the hardest of all, so we forget the kindness we show ourselves after a hard race. We even lament our new caregiving role on occasions, as it robs us of time to get part of our identity back. And if all the other women on social media can do it, then what's wrong with us? In frustration we blame everything around us, our babies, our food, our propensity for sitting on the sofa and eating another biscuit, our lack of motivation when the baby has a nap and so on and so on… This is the exact thought process I want to challenge so that we can move out of the guilt, regret, envy, shame, disappointment and pain and into a sense of realism that takes into account our new identity, respects our new priorities and sheds the excuses that worked for our old selves.

When you were asked to run for charity before you were a mother, all you had to do was perhaps leave work 20 minutes early to get in a quick training session before dinner. Priorities were so easily shifted, moved and adjusted. Now even toilet breaks can't be spontaneous! Prioritising your own exercise comes with a burden of guilt and the need for childcare[4-7]. This is by far the biggest challenge we must overcome as new mothers if we want to incorporate physical activity in our daily routines.

So why not start with ten (or five) squats at the top and bottom of the stairs whenever you need to go up and down? No time restrictions, no need to have any special kit or time getting ready. After a few weeks to a couple of months of this you will be getting fitter without much trying, and you will be able to build on this strength should you choose to do more specific activity later. Add whatever you feel you need to this basic training: planks for upper body strength, twists and stretches for flexibility. This 'bursts and starts' method of exercise has the same level of benefits if not more than any sustained moderate-intensity exercise such as a buggy walk or swim. So, don't miss these precious 10 to 30 seconds of time during your day. The numbers will soon stack up at the end of the day, week and month.

But I think exercising just to get physically stronger and sustain longer periods of activity is a rather limiting view of the health benefits of exercise in general. As physically active mums we have a better stress-response, counterintuitively experience less fatigue, and have better sleep quality than those who don't. We make better decisions, have better coordination, and are even keeping dementia at bay[8-10].

Once you feel more confident of your movements and want to build your exercise, you can join a class or two you enjoy. If you are going to a class, make sure your provider understands the postnatal life of a woman, not just the bodily changes. It is important you choose someone who is well versed in the physiology and biomechanics of a body that has recently given birth, but they should also be aware of how new mothers experience social pressures to get their 'pre-pregnancy body' back and help you navigate those thoughts in a sensitive and compassionate manner. At the moment there is no regulation or minimum qualification standard for class providers of antenatal and postnatal exercise. Don't be afraid to ask lots of questions, and go with your gut instinct and recommendations if you can.

Babywearing exercise

Also, realise that you don't have to exercise without your baby. A study looking at exercise sessions with or without babies reported more positive feelings when women exercised with their babies.[11] All mothers experienced the same benefits of reduced fatigue and reduced lower back pain, but the positive feelings among the women who exercised with their babies mean that they are more likely to adhere to exercise in future.

Babywearing exercise classes have become very popular in recent years. These classes, if structured correctly, can be a great source of shared experience for you and your baby. Moreover, you will discover other mothers who share your parenting style and these friendships will certainly motivate you to keep attending the class.

I started my babywearing yoga class when little Jessica was only seven weeks. What I enjoyed most was being among similarly minded new mothers who all knew the hardships of sleepless nights and social expectations. The class gave me and my baby precious time to be together without many distractions of toys and loud noises. We moved together, hummed together and mostly just hung out together. I really enjoyed slowing down. Rachael

The research on the benefits of babywearing is now robust, but the science of movement with babies in carriers, especially exercise, is still very patchy. Moreover, the many different types of carriers available make it even harder to translate research done on one type of carrier to another. It is important that all providers of babywearing exercise have training in the safety of babywearing and a basic understanding of movement principles of exercise with babies in slings and carriers. Some slings are more appropriate for exercise than others. You can consult your local sling library or your class provider about safe options.

Some general principles that will help you exercise safely with your baby in a carrier:

1. Carrying a baby changes your biomechanics of movement, whether in arms or in a carrier. If you carry your baby in front you are more likely to exaggerate your lumbar curve, and it also increases para-spinal muscle activation.[12,13]

This is compensatory mechanism to realign your centre of gravity and allow you to stay upright and mobile. In order that you don't injure or tire your lower back you need to wear the carrier nearer your waist and not lower near your hips. Try having baby as close (tight without squeezing) to your body as you can. The higher (across the whole of your trunk rather than your belly) and closer baby is to your body, the more efficient your movements will be. One study has shown that this simple adjustment can ensure your loaded movements (with baby) resemble your unloaded (no baby) movements.

2. This is important from a general fatigue perspective. If your baby is worn low (seat of the carrier down towards your belly/hips), you will round your upper back and close in your shoulders, which will dramatically reduce your breathing efficiency and also reduce your exercise capacity. Since you will be taking some of baby's weight passively over your shoulders, the shoulders may tire easily. Make sure your sling appropriately protects your shoulder and upper back posture and allows you to relax into the movements.

3. Carrying your baby higher and tighter will also protect your weakened pelvic floor. If you stay tall, taking most of the baby's weight on your trunk, your abdominal muscles will get stronger and take the load of the baby, which will reduce the burden on your pelvic floor.[12] This is especially important if you have even a mild prolapse. If your pelvic floor needs time to get stronger, wear your baby for shorter durations but do not completely stop (unless of course your healthcare professional advises you to). Doing small amounts of movement with a growing baby will allow you to understand how to hold baby's weight correctly from early days so that as they grow heavier it is not a big shock

to your system.

4. Appropriate breathing techniques are hugely important when it comes to babywearing exercise. In fact, I believe that not understanding breath mechanics will be more detrimental to your capacity and ability to enjoy babywearing exercise than any other aspect.

5. Breathing better will help you also to engage your core appropriately: protecting and strengthening your core, pelvic floor and other supporting tissues. Carriers tend to limit trunk flexion (folding forwards) and rotation, so good breathing techniques will come in handy when you do exercise. As a general rule, try to exhale on flexions and rotations.

There are also a few key points to consider with respect to your baby's movements when you exercise wearing them. First, it is important to consider all the safety points that are key to babywearing in general (the Carrying Matters website www.carryingmatters.co.uk is a great resource). Movement in slings bring further challenges. Keep a close eye on your baby's airway throughout your exercise, and at no point compromise their breathing for any manoeuvre/posture you may wish to do.

You need to adapt your exercise so that you do not put undue force on baby's neck and cervical spine. This means no jumping, no sprinting and no quick twirls. These movements will transfer the forces of your activity to your baby's undeveloped spine and create pressure which could lead to serious injury.[15]

Second, consider your baby's neck and head control. As you move, if your baby's neck is free to move too, they will feel your movements a lot faster than you feel them. Supporting their head and making sure their head is not moving independently of your movement counteracts this fast-moving feeling. Imagine your baby's head as a satellite of your own movement. Gently either hold your baby's head close to your body, or use the head support built into the carrier if there is one.

Finally, the principles of heat exertion for general exercise become even more important if you exercise with your baby in a sling. Your body heat will have less surface area to dissipate and the composition of your sling, environment and type of exercise you do will all factor into your hydration strategy.

By taking sensible precautions, exercising with your baby close to you can bring you both great rewards, including bonding, experiencing each other's non-verbal communication, and physiological co-regulatory benefits. As you share exercise you are helping them grow up finding physical movement something to enjoy, not endure.

One of the key things I learnt from doing babywearing yoga was how to have a good posture. The sling library was great in fitting the sling but after about an hour of walking my dog with my baby, I would find I was drooping in my posture and it gave me backache. Coming to the class (Babywearing yoga) helped me understand how to maintain my posture during all the activities as well as just standing. Louise

Exercise after caesarean

If you have had a caesarean section or assisted birth, please be extra mindful when starting to exercise. Assess your physical capacity on a regular basis and slow down when you need to. There is no evidence that says you cannot exercise a few weeks after a c-section[17,18]. Most guidance prudently suggests you wait until after your six-week check before embarking on a regimented exercise programme. However, physical activity has been shown to enhance recovery from all sorts of surgical procedures, and a sedentary lifestyle will lengthen your recovery time. So, move mindfully and slow down as soon as you recognise over-exertion.

> *As any woman who has experience of a c-section will know, the recovery is so long and hard. When I was pregnant, I was very active and stayed active till the end. So not being able to do much after my c-section is making me sad. I feel it is not just the birth, but my body needs the care and attention now more than ever before.* Elly

Perineal damage

Research indicates that one year after birth there is very little residual impact of the degree of perineal damage on pelvic muscle function. Exercise (specific pelvic floor or general physical activity) seems to be an outstanding contributor in regaining pelvic floor strength. More holistic, breath-modulated, strength and functional training has been shown to be instrumental in improving pelvic floor function and core stability, leading to improved range of movement. Please see detailed pelvic floor section in Chapter 8.

Diastasis recti

Diastasis recti is a condition identified as a gap of more than 2cm in the outermost layer of the abdominal muscles. This can be caused by intra-abdominal pressure during mid and late pregnancy, and may persist postnatally[19]. Good core strength, ligament flexibility and functional capacity are all required to maintain the integrity of the core muscles during pregnancy and help the abdominal muscle regain its structure and strength soon after birth. (See Chapter 8)

Thinking about your diet

As new mums our caring responsibilities often take precedence over self-care. This means we are can end up ignoring our need for nutritious food and instead relying on leftovers from under the highchair. No set meal times, no set hunger triggers, no control over nutrient consumption and little audit of total energy intake are a few possible issues that can mean you don't feel as good as you could. If you are breastfeeding your hormones trigger a hunger and craving pattern that may lead you to eat foods that have an unhealthy balance between carbohydrates and other nutrients that your body needs. If you would like to lose some body fat, making sure you eat enough to maintain your supply of breastmilk vs reducing fat-converting nutrients such as simple sugars should form part of your entire plan to get fitter. Ignoring food and prioritising exercise will lead to a lopsided effort and is a strategy for disappointment.

Cooking adult portions in batches and quickly warming them at mealtimes is one of the smartest food habits you can create. I also recommend a treat box. Put in the box only the treats you will eat in one day. That could be a couple of biscuits or a slice of cake or a few pieces of chocolate from a big bar. You can fill the box once a day, preferably after dinner (you won't be tempted to cheat if you do this on a full stomach). This habit saves you from two important energy-sapping problems: decision fatigue and sacrifice without a visible end point.

As a general rule, move before you eat. Aerobic and endurance exercises are best done in the morning after an overnight fast to allow for fat to mobilise much more quickly. Walks, runs and swims don't have to be hours long. A 15– 20 minute routine will give great benefits over time. This does not apply if you have any underlying metabolic issues, particularly diabetes or hypertension. Please be aware that exercise response can be very individual and if you have any concerns speak to your GP, midwife or even a professional exercise specialist who understands the perinatal period.

Weight management

Most of us, at some point in our postnatal life, start to think about our excess pregnancy weight. For some of us that question comes within days of giving birth and for some of us it remains in the background for months. I truly believe that there is no perfect time to start considering an exercise/food strategy, so don't feel guilty or pressured by external influences.

However, research[20] indicates that the longer we put off tackling this elephant in the room, the less likely it is that we will. The danger then is that you may enter subsequent pregnancies with this excess weight. The evidence links high BMI with increased birth complications, along with epigenetic implications for your baby.

When you feel ready to start considering weight management strategies, start slow and build up, to get more movement into your daily life. These simple strategies will help you build a unique lifestyle incorporating exercise and healthy eating patterns that will stay with you for life.

When thinking about weight management, it is important to focus on fat loss and retaining (or increasing) lean tissue rather than losing pounds on the scale. Lean tissue is several times heavier than body fat, so weight-loss strategies that focus on reducing body *weight* rather than body *fat* are unhelpful. Since lean mass is heavier and easier to lose with dieting you will see a reduction in your weight, but it won't be healthy in the long run. Also, once you lose lean mass it is very hard to gain back. So, make sure you include strength-based exercises in your plan.

Breastfeeding and losing weight

I am sure you have heard that you will lose weight if you breast feed, and this is not untrue. However, research indicates that the magnitude of weight loss is rather small if you rely only on the energetic cost of lactation to help you lose your excess body fat. Studies looking at over 36,000 Danish breastfeeding women reported lower weight retention only in women who were not overweight or obese. A similar study[21] of 14,300 women reported appreciable weight loss only if women exclusively breastfed for six months.

Energy requirements for breastfeeding are approximately 500kcal/day, so a concurrent increase in energy intake is recommended in the UK. This assumes that energy expenditure remains the same in the postnatal period as before pregnancy. However, most of us as new mothers find ourselves a lot more sedentary in the early days. This decrease in energy expenditure, coupled with an increase in energy intake for milk production, may prevent the expected weight loss. Studies looking at exercise and a small energy reduction in lactating mothers have clearly demonstrated that both exercise and diet are important for postnatal weight loss. If we add just exercise, we invariably compensate for that energy expenditure by simply increasing our intake. Since a small reduction in energy intake has been shown to have no impact on lactation, milk composition or weight gain and growth in infants, it is a strategy that can be applied sensibly.

However, if you find that you are feeling less energetic, your baby is not putting on weight or either of you are developing frequent upper respiratory tract infections such as colds and coughs, it is important to look at your energy intake, as low energy intake can cause your immune system to be less responsive.

Your exercise also alters your breastmilk composition. In one study[22], mice offspring from sedentary mothers were swapped 48 hours after birth to nurse with exercised rats and vice versa. The babies on breastmilk from exercised mothers had better glucose and insulin tolerance, and decreased fat and body weight compared to the offspring feeding from the sedentary mothers. Seven days after birth breastmilk from both sets of mice was analysed and the researchers found a certain key oligosaccharide (a type of non-digestible carbohydrate) in significantly higher amounts in breastmilk from exercised mothers compared to sedentary ones. When the researchers supplemented the breastmilk of sedentary mice with the oligosaccharide there was a significant improvement in glucose tolerance in the offspring.

Only initiate an energy-restricted diet and exercise programme once breastfeeding has been established. If possible, seek guidance from a professional lactation consultant/nutritionist and exercise professional to help you come up with a specific plan. Create a long-term sustainable plan rather a 'get back in my jeans for summer' plan.

Clothes

To accommodate both breastfeeding and exercise in your time-pressed day, you will want to be ready to exercise while being able to breast feed on demand. This is not straightforward, and there are many discussions about it on the internet. No matter how you decide to dress, make sure your bra is well-fitting and supportive of your extra sensitive breast tissue. Comfortable yoga-style clothing and thin layers that can be easily added and taken off may be useful.

I just used my maternity leggings in the postnatal period too! The elasticated pants were forgiving to all my extra weight and the stretch fabric was perfect for any exercise I would do without having to think too hard what to wear. Claire

Sisters in crime

Just as we humans enjoy a cup of coffee and cake with our friends, we also share our emotional state when we exercise together. Group activities have shown that dopamine (a neurotransmitter with a role in how we feel pleasure) is higher after an exercise session when participants exercised in a group compared to when they exercised on their own. If something feels good, we have an incentive to do it again.

Exercise alone improves mental health outcomes in new mothers, but social isolation can be a beast of its own. We may languish in our pyjamas as home, admonishing ourselves for not going out, unable to reach out to other supportive new mums who will share our mothering challenges. Group exercise can combat these feelings and forge new friendships.

Moving together has deeper benefits too. Our ancestors intuitively understood this and created rituals of dance and marching. New research[23,24] is catching up on the power of synchronicity in nature. Just as fireflies match their flashes when they fly in a group, humans fall in step with each other when they move together. This connection bonds us in a fundamental way. Groups that move together tend to cooperate, share resources and help each other in hard times – and this effect is of great benefit to new mothers.

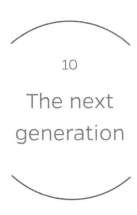

10

The next generation

Hopefully, the choices we make as parents will provide our children with lived examples rather than empty parental guidance. With this is mind, start involving your baby as early as you can in this positive practice of physical movement.

A series of infant sleep studies in the 1990s by researcher James McKenna[1] shows that parents and babies synchronise their breathing as part of their own collaborative way of communicating needs and physiological environments. Despite breathing rates being different, with babies breathing a lot faster, they show how sleep architecture follows a similar pattern in each mum and baby pair. This sense of connection carries on the more you hold your baby close. This is how our babies continue to learn from their mother's proximity, which is an extension of the uterine environment.

Slings and carriers are great tools for maternal breath and movement associations for newborn babies. As your breath dynamics change with your movement, your baby can gauge your physical and emotional state[2]. Long, elongated exhalations that excite your parasympathetic nervous system make the baby calmer too as they sense that you are calm and they are safe.

> *I know Roby knows when he gets in the sling with me it is going to be rest time. He is not even a couple of months, but I am amazed at how astute babies are. I have always created a gentle environment for him, singing, swaying and moving without too many distractions. I take these moments when I am putting him to sleep for myself too. I practice my breathing slowly and feel it's not just him, but I get rest too. It's a ritual now and putting him to sleep is something I look forward to, retreating in a room or a corner being by ourselves.* Anabelle

Your baby can also feel the vibrations of your voice and breath through your chest as they stay cosy in the sling. If you embody the principles of correct posture, understanding the constant shifts in centre of gravity as you move with your baby in a sling or carrier, this can be a profound experiential practice to pass on to your baby.

This also means your baby does not have sit it out when you exercise: they come along, they know the importance of movement in your life, and they naturally want to emulate this habit themselves.

The mother-baby dyad

The foundations of parent-child relationships are established in early infancy. If these relationships involve positive role-modelling and secure attachment, our children learn behavioural and emotional self-regulation as they grow up. Robust research[3] shows that insecure attachment in babies 15, 24 and 36 months of age correlates strongly with odds of obesity at 15 years. This makes sense, as secure attachment influences stress response, appetite, sleep and long-term self-regulation. All these are important aspects of weight management and health outcomes in children as they grow.

Some current research[4] indicates that a mother's dissatisfaction with her body during pregnancy and the postnatal period can have a subtle yet profound impact on her mental health, which then affects her relationship with her baby. Being physically active certainly makes us feel better, but body dissatisfaction can be an issue whether you exercise or not. It is thus important to pay attention to positive role models, meaningful social influences and internal positive dialogues to regulate our feelings about our body and monitor our psychological health.

By modelling behaviours and choices for our babies from an early age, along with creating secure bonds, we pave the way for our babies to grow up with a positive body image, healthy relationship with food and exercise and to view exercise from a health and wellbeing perspective rather than a simplistic weight management perspective. It is these subtle yet profound shifts in our own relationship with physical exercise and movement that will help us pass it on to the next generation

Exercise and the family

A family that exercises together, stays lean together! Even though I have spun this phrase around, the evidence supports it. Research[5-10] into how best to engage children to combat childhood obesity indicates that interventions that include the whole family are more likely to create sustainable habits than those targeted at children alone. On the flip side, if a child has one parent who is overweight or obese, then their chances of becoming obese are 28% compared to 8% for children who have a parent of normal weight. However, if both the child's parents are obese then their own chances of becoming obese are a whopping 60%[5].

A meta-analysis[7] has shown that family support and attitudes to exercise within the family have a much larger effect on actual behaviour than most other areas of influence. Thus, if we move beyond the perinatal period, we need to embrace a lifestyle that will allow our whole family to live in an active way. This could mean engaging in age-appropriate physical activities and finding new ways to enjoy moving more as a family. Of course, the grounding that a beautiful solitary jog or swim brings has immense benefits for our physical and mental wellbeing, but we need to be actively engaging our children in our passion for physical activity.

Many households try to spend mealtimes together, but the parents still go out to exercise on their own. This is sometimes due to the logistics of childcare, and sometimes due to the nature of the activity itself. They then take the kids to their own activity sessions separately. From a family perspective this model may be practical, but it does mean that our habits of staying active might not be as visible to our children, who may experience your time at the gym or yoga class as time away from them. If you can arrange to do a few activities that can be enjoyed by the whole family, you are more likely to help your children make exercise habits an integral part of their life. A bit like brushing their teeth!

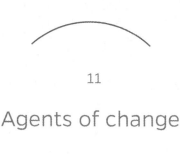

11

Agents of change

Healthcare providers can be influential agents of change at one of the most pivotal points in the lives of women. There is no other time in our lives when our bodies, lifestyles and priorities undergo such a dramatic and obvious upheaval than the perinatal period. Data suggests that even in normal circumstances people are seven times more likely to go to an exercise class and 12 times more likely to become more physically active when the suggestion comes from a professional quarter.[1] At a time when we are all recognising the importance of physical, mental and emotional health in our chances of getting pregnant, having a fulfilling pregnancy and reducing risks at birth, our care providers have an amazing golden opportunity to engage us in a more active lifestyle. Yet 72% of GPs do not recommend physical activity to their patients (not just pregnant and new mothers). Key barriers are a lack of knowledge, confidence and resources.[2]

In 2016, the Better Births[3] report identified the need for meaningful conversations with our care providers on physical activity: '*each woman needs to engage in a relationship with her own midwife and other health professionals, acting on advice where she can make a difference, e.g., by accepting help to give up smoking, having a healthy diet and being physically active*' (pp.84-85).

Therefore, midwives have a particularly important role. In a recent study,[4] midwives who were interviewed identified a lack of specific knowledge and training on giving exercise advice and guidance to the people in their care. They also said that physical activity was a 'tick box' for the booking appointment, and that there are no recurring prompts to discuss physical activity during antenatal care.

Many midwives have identified a lack of knowledge and support as barriers to discussing physical activity with the women in their care. Antenatal care teams may have specialist dietitians who can advise on food intake for women who need extra support. But we do not have qualified exercise specialists who know the nuances of pregnancy and postnatal exercise requirements. This omission has caused many midwives and other care providers to shoulder the responsibility for promoting physical activity to pregnant and new mothers. Unfortunately, this leads to advice that can be generic, laden with personal bias and preferences and that can cause a sense of anxiety in professionals who are not trained in exercise.

One study[5] of midwives involved in teaching aquanatal classes in the North-West asked how they felt about teaching the class. Only half of the respondents felt they were ideal for the job. Not everyone taking the class was given training for it, and of those who were trained, many felt that the training was not adequate.

I was forever asking the midwives [about exercise activities] but I got swapped between a few midwives... so I kind of found out there wasn't much information out there. Rachel

Some of the more insidious reasons midwives have given for not talking about physical activity during pregnancy include fear of litigation, high workload and their own personal beliefs.

I don't think a pregnant woman is going to start exercising because she is pregnant necessarily. Anne[4]

Midwives under this sort of pressure will struggle to help women feel confident about starting or continuing to be active during pregnancy.

One way around the problem is to consider other areas of public health and identify pockets of good practice that can be borrowed to improve physical activity in pregnancy and postnatal period. For example, the WHO framework[6] on smoking cessation, the '5As' (Ask, Assess, Advise, Agree, Assist), has been used successfully in many fields. It could be a simple yet effective conversation starter in antenatal and postnatal clinics, to address the topic of physical activity.

However, it is not enough to just start the conversation – it is important to keep the momentum going. Without a commitment to support women becoming and staying active throughout their lives, it will inevitably fall by the wayside.

In the UK we have amazing exercise science expertise. However, we need to focus this expertise on the perinatal period of our lives, as it is not just about serving women, but also getting it right for our future generations. The health impact, the long-term financial benefit to our health services and a collective culture of being active across all age groups starts with mothers and the babies in their wombs.

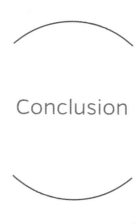

Conclusion

My hope is that this book will have given you a reason to move more, some confidence and some first steps. We live in times where inspiration and motivation can come from any corner, not just experts or celebrities. Our democratic way of sharing knowledge means we can all support each other in doing a bit more physical activity and inspire each other on days when we are less motivated.

If you want to encourage other pregnant and new mothers and find encouragement for yourself, do engage in our ongoing conversation using the hashtag #MoveMoreMum.

I also hope that the evidence presented here will convince our healthcare providers of the need to prescribe more activity to pregnant women and new mothers. The impact of incorporating a physical activity pathway in all pregnancy care packages, not just high-risk categories, is hugely important.

We need more than posters and prompts.

Us mothers who are growing and raising future generations need support and resources to ensure that being less sedentary is not simply a responsibility dumped on us as individuals, further adding to the long list of things we already have on our plates. We need all the relevant stakeholders: employers, childcare systems and the government, to cooperate in making physical activity a sustainable lifestyle choice during pregnancy and the postnatal period.

Acknowledgements

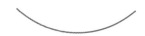

This book started with a personal passion, but has been made possible by the pregnant women and new mothers I have met in the last few years. Many echoed my tentative worries about exercise in early pregnancy, and many new mothers lamented the lack of support and guidance available to help them stay active. I felt compelled to write this book because of you. Thank you for your open and honest conversations.

Finding time to write was a real challenge, and here I must thank Rees, my partner. His incredible belief in my ability to write this book, his generosity with his time, patience and his ability to make me even more coffee are probably the reasons I finished the book. I also thank Rees for drawing the explanatory diagrams. I must of course mention my three daughters. Despite being only five and three my older girls understood this was important to me and it was extra special to write this book whilst being pregnant with my third.

I also thank the teachers I have had the privilege to learn from: Kaizzad, Leslie, Michel, Lous and so many of you that I haven't named.

Finally, my biggest thanks go to the team at Pinter & Martin, for giving me the opportunity. Zoë, Susan and Martin, thank you for making this experience so positive and for your support, clear guidance and encouragement.

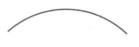

References

Chapter 1: A brief history of pregnancy and postnatal exercise

1. Chavasse, P. H. (1844). Advice to Wives on the Management of Themselves: During the Periods of Pregnancy, Labour, and Suckling. D. Appleton.
2. Karamanou, M., Tsoucalas, G., Creatsas, G., & Androutsos, G. (2013). The effect of Soranus of Ephesus (98–138) on the work of midwives. Women and Birth
3. Browne, F. J. (1939). Antenatal and postnatal care. The Lancet, 234(6066), 1192.
4. Bruser, M. (1968). Sporting Activities during pregnancy. Obstetrics & Gynecology: Volume 32 - Issue 5 - p 721-725.
5. Davies, G. A., Wolfe, L. A., Mottola, M. F., & MacKinnon, C. (2003). Joint SOGC/CSEP clinical practice guideline: exercise in pregnancy and the postpartum period. Canadian Journal of Applied Physiology, 28(3), 329-341.
6. Harrison, A. L., Taylor, N. F., Shields, N., & Frawley, H. C. (2018). Attitudes, barriers and enablers to physical activity in pregnant women: a systematic review. Journal of Physiotherapy, 64(1).
7. Jawadwala, R. (2019) Want to get moving? AIMS Journal, 2019, Vol 31, No 3 ISSN 2516-5852
8. Mottola, M. F., Davenport, M. H., Ruchat, S.-M., Davies, G. A., Poitras, V. J., Gray, C. E., … Zehr, L. (2018). 2019 Canadian guideline for physical activity throughout pregnancy. British Journal of Sports Medicine, 52(21), 1339.

Overview reading:

Kehler, A. K., & Heinrich, K. M. (2015). A selective review of prenatal exercise guidelines since the 1950s until present: Written for women, health care professionals, and female athletes. *Women and Birth*. Elsevier.

Chapter 2: A dramatic transformation

1. Gilleard W.L. (2018) Increased Step Width During Walking as Pregnancy Progresses: Functional or Mechanical Adaptation?. In: Brandão S., Da Roza T., Ramos I., Mascarenhas T. (eds) Women's Health and Biomechanics. Lecture Notes in Computational Vision and Biomechanics, vol 29. Springer, Cham

2. Liddle, S. D., & Pennick, V. (2015). Interventions for preventing and treating low-back and pelvic pain during pregnancy. *Cochrane Database of Systematic Reviews*.

3. Jang, J., Hsiao, K. T., & Hsiao-Wecksler, E. T. (2008). Balance (perceived and actual) and preferred stance width during pregnancy. *Clinical Biomechanics*, 23(4), 468–476.

4. Clapp III, J. F., Seaward, B. L., Sleamaker, R. H., & Hiser, J. (1988). Maternal physiologic adaptations to early human pregnancy. *American journal of obstetrics and gynecology*, 159(6), 1456-1460.

5. May, L. (2015). Cardiac physiology of pregnancy. *Comprehensive Physiology*, 5(3), 1325–1344.

6. Beetham, K. S., Giles, C., Noetel, M., Clifton, V., Jones, J. C., & Naughton, G. (2019). The effects of vigorous intensity exercise in the third trimester of pregnancy: a systematic review and meta-analysis. *BMC Pregnancy and Childbirth*, 19(1), 281.

7. Ferraro, Z. M., Chaput, J.-P., Gruslin, A., & Adamo, K. B. (2014). The Potential Value of Sleep Hygiene for a Healthy Pregnancy: A Brief Review. *ISRN Family Medicine*, 2014, 1–7.

8. Reichner, C. A. (2015). Insomnia and sleep deficiency in pregnancy. *Obstetric medicine*, 8(4), 168-171.

9. Lee, K. A., & Gay, C. L. (2004). Sleep in late pregnancy predicts length of labor and type of delivery. *American journal of obstetrics and gynecology*, 191(6), 2041-2046.

10. Kredlow, M. A., Capozzoli, M. C., Hearon, B. A., Calkins, A. W., & Otto, M. W. (2015). The effects of physical activity on sleep: a meta-analytic review. *Journal of behavioral medicine*, 38(3), 427-449.

11. Miller, B. H., Olson, S. L., Turek, F. W., Levine, J. E., Horton, T. H., & Takahashi, J. S. (2004). Circadian clock mutation disrupts estrous cyclicity and maintenance of pregnancy. *Current biology : CB*, 14(15), 1367–1373.

Overview reading:

Chang, J., & Streitman, D. (2012). Physiologic Adaptations to Pregnancy. *Neurologic Clinics*, 30(3), 781–789.

Chapter 3: Ways to incorporate physical activity

1. Perales, M., Santos-Lozano, A., Ruiz, J. R., Lucia, A., & Barakat, R. (2016). Benefits of aerobic or resistance training during pregnancy on maternal health and perinatal outcomes: A systematic review. *Early Human Development*, *94*, 43–48.

2. Kuhrt, K., Harmon, M., Hezelgrave, N. L., Seed, P. T., & Shennan, A. H. (2018). Is recreational running associated with earlier delivery and lower birth weight in women who continue to run during pregnancy? An international retrospective cohort study of running habits of 1293 female runners during pregnancy. *BMJ Open Sport Exerc Med*, *4*, 296.

3. https://assets.publishing.service.gov.uk/government/uploads/system/uploads/attachment_data/file/829894/5-physical-activity-for-pregnant-women.pdf

4. Salvesen, K. Å., Hem, E., & Sundgot-Borgen, J. (2012). Fetal wellbeing may be compromised during strenuous exercise among pregnant elite athletes. *British journal of sports medicine*, *46*(4), 279–283.

5. de Barros, M. C., Lopes, M. A., Francisco, R. P., Sapienza, A. D., & Zugaib, M. (2010). Resistance exercise and glycemic control in women with gestational diabetes mellitus. *American journal of obstetrics and gynecology*, *203*(6), 556-e1.

6. Barakat, R., & Perales, M. (2016). Resistance Exercise in Pregnancy and Outcome. *Clinical obstetrics and gynecology*, *59*(3), 591–599.

7. Di Biase, N., Balducci, S., Lencioni, C., Bertolotto, A., Tumminia, A., Dodesini, A. R., … Napoli, A. (2019). Review of general suggestions on physical activity to prevent and treat gestational and pre-existing diabetes during pregnancy and in postpartum. *Nutrition, Metabolism and Cardiovascular Diseases*. Elsevier B.V.

8. Skow, R. J., Davenport, M. H., Mottola, M. F., Davies, G. A., Poitras, V. J., Gray, C. E., ... & Adamo, K. B. (2019). Effects of prenatal exercise on fetal heart rate, umbilical and uterine blood flow: a systematic review and meta-analysis. *British journal of sports medicine*, *53*(2), 124-133.

9. Silveira, C., Pereira, B. G., Cecatti, J. G., Cavalcante, S. R., & Pereira, R. I. (2010). Fetal cardiotocography before and after water aerobics during pregnancy. *Reproductive Health*, *7*(1), 23.

10. Katz, V. L. (1996). *Water Exercise in Pregnancy*.

11. Katz, V. L., McMurray, R., Goodwin, W. E., & Cefalo, R. C. (1990). Non weight bearing exercise during pregnancy on land and during immersion: a comparative study. *American journal of perinatology*, *7*(3), 281–284.

12. Katz, V. L., McMurray, R., Berry, M. J., & Cefalo, R. C. (1988). Fetal and uterine responses to immersion and exercise. *Obstetrics and gynecology*, *72*(2), 225-230.

13. Juhl, Mettea; Kogevinas, Manolisb,c,d,e; Andersen, Per Kraghf; Andersen, Anne-Marie Nybog; Olsen, Jørnh Is Swimming During Pregnancy a Safe Exercise?, Epidemiology: March 2010 - Volume 21 - Issue 2 - p 253-258

14. Nieuwenhuijsen, M. J., Toledano, M. B., Eaton, N. E., Fawell, J., & Elliott, P. (2000). Chlorination disinfection byproducts in water and their association with adverse reproductive outcomes: a review. *Occupational and environmental medicine, 57*(2), 73–85.

15. Agopian, A. J., Lupo, P. J., Canfield, M. A., Mitchell, L. E., & Study, N. B. D. P. (2013). Swimming pool use and birth defect risk. *American Journal of Obstetrics and Gynecology, 209*(3), 219-e1.

16. Babbar, S., Parks-Savage, A., & Chauhan, S. (2012). Yoga during Pregnancy: A Review- Google Scholar. *American Journal of Perinatology …, 29*(6), 459–464.

17. de Campos, E. A., Narchi, N. Z., & Moreno, G. (2020). Meanings and perceptions of women regarding the practice of yoga in pregnancy: A qualitative study. *Complementary Therapies in Clinical Practice, 39*.

18. Narendran, S., Nagarathna, R., Narendran, V., Gunasheela, S., & Rama Rao Nagendra, H. (2005). Efficacy of yoga on pregnancy outcome. *Journal of Alternative and Complementary Medicine*

19. Beddoe, A. E., Paul Yang, C. P., Kennedy, H. P., Weiss, S. J., & Lee, K. A. (2009). The effects of mindfulness-based yoga during pregnancy on maternal psychological and physical distress. *JOGNN - Journal of Obstetric, Gynecologic, and Neonatal Nursing.*

20. Kwon, R., Kasper, K., London, S., & Haas, D. M. (2020). A systematic review: The effects of yoga on pregnancy. European Journal of Obstetrics & Gynecology and Reproductive Biology.

21. Mohyadin, E., Ghorashi, Z., & Molamomanaei, Z. (2020). The effect of practicing yoga during pregnancy on labor stages length, anxiety and pain: a randomized controlled trial. Journal of Complementary and Integrative Medicine, 1(ahead-of-print).

22. Russo, M. A., Santarelli, D. M., & O'Rourke, D. (2017, December 1). The physiological effects of slow breathing in the healthy human. *Breathe*. European Respiratory Society.

23. Busch, V., Magerl, W., Kern, U., Haas, J., Hajak, G., & Eichhammer, P. (2012). The effect of deep and slow breathing on pain perception, autonomic activity, and mood processing—an experimental study. *Pain Medicine, 13*(2), 215-228.

Overview reading:

Coll, C. V., Domingues, M. R., Gonçalves, H., & Bertoldi, A. D. (2017). Perceived barriers to leisure-time physical activity during pregnancy: A literature review of quantitative and qualitative evidence. Journal of science and medicine in sport, 20(1), 17-25.

Chapter 4: How much exercise is enough?

1. Preston, J. D., Reynolds, L. J., & Pearson, K. J. (2018, March 1). Developmental Origins of Health Span and Life Span: A Mini-Review. *Gerontol-*

ogy. S. Karger AG.

2. Acosta-Manzano, P., Acosta, F. M., Femia, P., Coll-Risco, I., Segura-Jiménez, V., Díaz-Castro, J., ... Aparicio, V. A. (2020). Association of sedentary time and physical activity levels with immune metabolic markers in early pregnancy: The GESTAFIT project. *Scandinavian Journal of Medicine & Science in Sports*, 30(1), 148–158.

3. Clapp III, J. F., & Kiess, W. (2000). Effects of pregnancy and exercise on concentrations of the metabolic markers tumor necrosis factor α and leptin. *American journal of obstetrics and gynecology*, 182(2), 300-306.

4. Edwards, M. J. (1967). Congenital defects in guinea-pigs following induced hyperthermia during gestation. *Arch Pathol*, 84, 42-48.

5. Edwards, M. J. (1968). Congenital malformations in the rat following induced hyperthermia during gestation. *Teratology*, 1(2), 173-177.

6. Edwards, M. J. (1969). Congenital defects in guinea pigs: fetal resorptions, abortions, and malformations following induced hyperthermia during early gestation. *Teratology*, 2(4), 313-328.

7. Uhari, M., Mustonen, A., & Kouvalainen, K. (1979). Sauna habits of Finnish women during pregnancy. *British medical journal*, 1(6172), 1216.

8. Ravanelli, N., Casasola, W., English, T., Edwards, K. M., & Jay, O. (2019). Heat stress and fetal risk. Environmental limits for exercise and passive heat stress during pregnancy: a systematic review with best evidence synthesis. *British journal of sports medicine*, 53(13), 799-805.

Overview reading:

Mudd, L. M., Owe, K. M., Mottola, M. F., & Pivarnik, J. M. (2013). Health benefits of physical activity during pregnancy: an international perspective. Med Sci Sports Exerc, 45(2), 268-77.

Chapter 5: Exercise and nutrition

1. Chang, T., Ravi, N., Pleque, M. A., Sonneville, K. R., & Davis, M. M. (2016). Inadequate hydration, BMI, and obesity among US adults: NHANES 2009–2012. *The Annals of Family Medicine*, 14(4), 320-324.

2. Zhang, N., Zhang, F., Chen, S., Han, F., Lin, G., Zhai, Y., ... & Ma, G. (2020). Associations between hydration state and pregnancy complications, maternal-infant outcomes: protocol of a prospective observational cohort study. *BMC pregnancy and childbirth*, 20(1), 82.

3. Ndikom, C. M., Fawole, B., & Ilesanmi, R. E. (2014). Extra fluids for breastfeeding mothers for increasing milk production. *Cochrane Database of Systematic Reviews*, (6).

4. Kominiarek, M. A., & Rajan, P. (2016). Nutrition Recommendations in Pregnancy and Lactation. *The Medical Clinics of North America*, 100(6), 1199–1215.

5. Clapp III, J. F. (2002). Maternal carbohydrate intake and pregnancy outcome. *Proceedings of the Nutrition Society*, 61(1), 45–50.

6. Edwards, S. M., Cunningham, S. A., Dunlop, A. L., & Corwin, E. J. (2017). The Maternal Gut Microbiome during Pregnancy. *MCN The American Journal of Maternal/Child Nursing*, *42*(6), 310–316.

7. Sudo, N., Chida, Y., Aiba, Y., Sonoda, J., Oyama, N., Yu, X. N., ... & Koga, Y. (2004). Postnatal microbial colonization programs the hypothalamic–pituitary–adrenal system for stress response in mice. *The Journal of physiology*, *558*(1), 263-275.

8. Komaroff, A. L. (2017). The microbiome and risk for obesity and diabetes. *Jama*, *317*(4), 355-356.

9. Rakers, F., Rupprecht, S., Dreiling, M., Bergmeier, C., Witte, O. W., & Schwab, M. (2017). Transfer of maternal psychosocial stress to the fetus. *Neuroscience & Biobehavioral Reviews*.

10. Beijers, R., Buitelaar, J. K., & de Weerth, C. (2014). Mechanisms underlying the effects of prenatal psychosocial stress on child outcomes: beyond the HPA axis. *European child & adolescent psychiatry*, *23*(10), 943-956.

11. Bressa, C., Bailén-Andrino, M., Pérez-Santiago, J., González-Soltero, R., Pérez, M., Montalvo-Lominchar, M. G., ... & Larrosa, M. (2017). Differences in gut microbiota profile between women with active lifestyle and sedentary women. *PLoS One*, *12*(2), e0171352.

12. Mach, N., & Fuster-Botella, D. (2017). Endurance exercise and gut microbiota: A review. *Journal of Sport and Health Science*, *6*(2), 179-197.

Overview reading:

Singh, S. B., Madan, J., Coker, M., Hoen, A., Baker, E. R., Karagas, M. R., & Mueller, N. T. (2020). Does birth mode modify associations of maternal pre-pregnancy BMI and gestational weight gain with the infant gut microbiome? *International Journal of Obesity*, *44*(1), 23–32.

Chapter 6: Preparing for the physicality of birth

1. Dunn, P.M. (1989). Francois Mauriceau (1637-1709) and maternal posture for parturition. *Archives of disease in childhood*, 66 1 Spec No, 78-9 .

2. Liu, Y. C. (1979). Position during labor and delivery: History and perspective. *Journal of Nurse-Midwifery*, *24*(3), 23–26

3. Thurber, C., Dugas, L. R., Ocobock, C., Carlson, B., Speakman, J. R., & Pontzer, H. (2019). Extreme events reveal an alimentary limit on sustained maximal human energy expenditure. *Science advances*, *5*(6).

4. Soehnchen, N., Melzer, K., de Tejada, B. M., Jastrow-Meyer, N., Othenin-Girard, V., Irion, O., ... & Kayser, B. (2011). Maternal heart rate changes during labour. *European journal of obstetrics & gynecology and reproductive biology*, *158*(2), 173-178.

5. Whitburn, L. Y., Jones, L. E., Davey, M. A., & McDonald, S. (2019). The nature of labour pain: An updated review of the literature. *Women and Birth*. Elsevier B.V.

6. Farley, D., Piszczek, Ł., & Bąbel, P. (2019). Why is running a marathon

like giving birth? The possible role of oxytocin in the underestimation of the memory of pain induced by labor and intense exercise. *Medical Hypotheses*, *128*, 86–90.

7. Davenport, M. H., Ruchat, S. M., Sobierajski, F., Poitras, V. J., Gray, C. E., Yoo, C., Skow, R. J., Jaramillo Garcia, A., Barrowman, N., Meah, V. L., Nagpal, T. S., Riske, L., James, M., Nuspl, M., Weeks, A., Marchand, A. A., Slater, L. G., Adamo, K. B., Davies, G. A., Barakat, R., ... Mottola, M. F. (2019). Impact of prenatal exercise on maternal harms, labour and delivery outcomes: a systematic review and meta-analysis. *British journal of sports medicine*, *53*(2), 99–107.

8. White, E., Pivarnik, J., & Pfeiffer, K. (2014). Resistance training during pregnancy and perinatal outcomes. *Journal of Physical Activity and Health*.

9. Baciuk, E. P., Pereira, R. I., Cecatti, J. G., Braga, A. F., & Cavalcante, S. R. (2008). Water aerobics in pregnancy: cardiovascular response, labor and neonatal outcomes. *Reproductive Health*, *5*(1), 10.

10. Rodríguez-Blanque, R., Sánchez-García, J. C., Sánchez-López, A. M., & Aguilar-Cordero, M. J. (2019). Physical activity during pregnancy and its influence on delivery time: a randomized clinical trial. *PeerJ*, *7*, e6370–e6370.

11. Kardel, K. R., Johansen, B., Voldner, N., Iversen, P. O., & Henriksen, T. (2009). Association between aerobic fitness in late pregnancy and duration of labor in nulliparous women. *Acta obstetricia et gynecologica Scandinavica*, *88*(8), 948-952.

12. Dias, Letícia A. R., Driusso, Patricia, Aita, Daniella L. C. C., Quintana, Silvana M., Bø, Kari, & Ferreira, Cristine H. J.. (2011). Effect of pelvic floor muscle training on labour and newborn outcomes: a randomized controlled trial. *Brazilian Journal of Physical Therapy*, *15*(6), 487-493. Epub August 19, 2011.

13. Agur, W., Steggles, P., Waterfield, M., & Freeman, R. (2008). Does antenatal pelvic floor muscle training affect the outcome of labour? A randomised controlled trial. *International Urogynecology Journal*, *19*(1), 85–88.

14. Mette, J. (2009). *Physical exercise during pregnancy and reproductive outcomes*. University of Copenhagen.

15. Owe, K. M., Nystad, W., Stigum, H., Vangen, S., & Bø, K. (2016). Exercise during pregnancy and risk of cesarean delivery in nulliparous women: a large population-based cohort study. In *American Journal of Obstetrics and Gynecology*.

16. Silveira, L. C. da, & Segre, C. A. de M. (2012). Physical exercise during pregnancy and its influence in the type of birth. *Einstein (São Paulo, Brazil)*.

17. Morgan, K. L., Rahman, M. A., Hill, R. A., Zhou, S.-M., Bijlsma, G., Khanom, A., ... Brophy, S. T. (2014). Physical Activity and Excess Weight in Pregnancy Have Independent and Unique Effects on Delivery and Perina-

tal Outcomes. *PLoS ONE, 9*(4), e94532.

18. Poyatos-León, R., García-Hermoso, A., Sanabria-Martínez, G., Álvarez-Bueno, C., Sánchez-López, M., & Martínez-Vizcaíno, V. (2015). Effects of exercise during pregnancy on mode of delivery: A meta-analysis. *Acta Obstetricia et Gynecologica Scandinavica*.

19. Hartmann, S., & Bung, P. (1999). Physical exercise during pregnancy - Physiological considerations and recommendations. *Journal of Perinatal Medicine, 27*(3), 204–215.

20. Kabiru, W., & Raynor, B. D. (2004). Obstetric outcomes associated with increase in BMI category during pregnancy. *American journal of obstetrics and gynecology, 191*(3), 928-932.

21. Huang, L., Fan, L., Ding, P., He, Y. H., Xie, C., Niu, Z., ... & Chen, W. Q. (2018). The mediating role of placenta in the relationship between maternal exercise during pregnancy and full-term low birth weight. *The Journal of Maternal-Fetal & Neonatal Medicine, 31*(12), 1561-1567.

22. Evenson, K. R., Siega-Riz, A. M., Savitz, D. A., Leiferman, J. A., & Thorp Jr, J. M. (2002). Vigorous leisure activity and pregnancy outcome. *Epidemiology, 13*(6), 653-659.

23. Mette, J. (2009). *Physical exercise during pregnancy and reproductive outcomes*. University of Copenhagen.

Overview reading:

Michalek, I. M., Comte, C., & Desseauve, D. (2020). Impact of maternal physical activity during an uncomplicated pregnancy on fetal and neonatal well-being parameters: a systematic review of the literature. European Journal of Obstetrics & Gynecology and Reproductive Biology.

Chapter 7: How your unborn baby responds to exercise

1. Clapp III, J. F. (2003). The effects of maternal exercise on fetal oxygenation and feto-placental growth. *European Journal of Obstetrics & Gynecology and Reproductive Biology, 110*, S80-S85.

2. Clapp III, J. F., Kim, H., Burciu, B., & Lopez, B. (2000). Beginning regular exercise in early pregnancy: effect on fetoplacental growth. *American journal of obstetrics and gynecology, 183*(6), 1484-1488.

3. Beetham, K. S., Giles, C., Noetel, M., Clifton, V., Jones, J. C., & Naughton, G. (2019). The effects of vigorous intensity exercise in the third trimester of pregnancy: a systematic review and meta-analysis. *BMC pregnancy and childbirth, 19*(1), 281.

4. Skow, R. J., Davenport, M. H., Mottola, M. F., Davies, G. A., Poitras, V. J., Gray, C. E., ... & Adamo, K. B. (2019). Effects of prenatal exercise on fetal heart rate, umbilical and uterine blood flow: a systematic review and meta-analysis. *British journal of sports medicine, 53*(2), 124-133.

5. Webb, K. A., Wolfe, L. A., & McGrath, M. J. (1994). Effects of acute and chronic maternal exercise on fetal heart rate. *Journal of applied physiolo-*

gy, *77*(5), 2207-2213.

6. Velazquez, M. A., Fleming, T. P., & Watkins, A. J. (2019). Periconceptional environment and the developmental origins of disease. *Journal of Endocrinology*. BioScientifica Ltd.

7. Badon, S. E., Littman, A. J., Chan, K. C. G., Tadesse, M. G., Stapleton, P. L., Bammler, T. K., … Enquobahrie, D. A. (2018). Physical activity and epigenetic biomarkers in maternal blood during pregnancy. *Epigenomics*, *10*(11), 1383–1395.

8. Gluckman, P. D., Hanson, M. A., Cooper, C., & Thornburg, K. L. (2008, July 3). Effect of in utero and early-life conditions on adult health and disease. *New England Journal of Medicine*. Massachussetts Medical Society.

9. Juhl, M., Olsen, J., Andersen, P. K., Nøhr, E. A., & Andersen, A. M. N. (2010). Physical exercise during pregnancy and fetal growth measures: a study within the Danish National Birth Cohort. *American journal of obstetrics and gynecology*, *202*(1), 63-e1.

10. Fleten, C., Stigum, H., Magnus, P., & Nystad, W. (2010). Exercise during pregnancy, maternal prepregnancy body mass index, and birth weight. *Obstetrics & Gynecology*, *115*(2), 331-337.

11. Clapp III, J. F., & Capeless, E. L. (1990). Neonatal morphometrics after endurance exercise during pregnancy. *American journal of obstetrics and gynecology*, *163*(6), 1805-1811.

12. Haire-Joshu, D., & Tabak, R. (2016). Preventing Obesity Across Generations: Evidence for Early Life Intervention. *Annual Review of Public Health*, *37*(1), 253–271.

13. Xu, W. H., Wu, H., Xia, W. L., Lan, H., Wang, Y., Zhang, Y., & Hua, S. (2017). Physical exercise before pregnancy helps the development of mouse embryos produced in vitro. *Mitochondrion*, *34*, 36–42.

14. Mottola, M. F., & Artal, R. (2016). Fetal and maternal metabolic responses to exercise during pregnancy. *Early human development*, *94*, 33-41.

15. Clapp III, J. F. (1996). Morphometric and neurodevelopmental outcome at age five years of the offspring of women who continued to exercise regularly throughout pregnancy. *The Journal of pediatrics*, *129*(6), 856-863.

16. Clapp III, J. F., Simonian, S., Lopez, B., Appleby-Wineberg, S., & Harcar-Sevcik, R. (1998). The one-year morphometric and neurodevelopmental outcome of the offspring of women who continued to exercise regularly throughout pregnancy. *American journal of obstetrics and gynecology*, *178*(3), 594-599.

17. Domingues, M. R., Matijasevich, A., Barros, A. J., Santos, I. S., Horta, B. L., & Hallal, P. C. (2014). Physical activity during pregnancy and offspring neurodevelopment and IQ in the first 4 years of life. PloS one, 9(10), e110050.

18. Ferrari, N., Bae-Gartz, I., Bauer, C., Janoschek, R., Koxholt, I., Mahabir, E., … Graf, C. (2018). Exercise during pregnancy and its impact on mothers and offspring in humans and mice. *Journal of Developmental Origins of Health and Disease*, *9*(1), 63–76.

19. Laker, R. C., Wlodek, M. E., Connelly, J. J., & Yan, Z. (2013). Epigenetic origins of metabolic disease: the impact of the maternal condition to the offspring epigenome and later health consequences. *Food Science and Human Wellness*, 2(1), 1-11.

20. Preston, J. D., Reynolds, L. J., & Pearson, K. J. (2018). Developmental origins of health span and life span: a mini-review. *Gerontology*, 64(3), 237-245.

21. Melnik, B. C., & Schmitz, G. (2017). Milk's role as an epigenetic regulator in health and disease. *Diseases*, 5(1), 12.

22. Gabbianelli, R., Bordoni, L., Morano, S., Calleja-Agius, J., & Lalor, J. G. (2020). Nutri-Epigenetics and Gut Microbiota: How Birth Care, Bonding and Breastfeeding Can Influence and Be Influenced?. *International Journal of Molecular Sciences*, 21(14), 5032.

Overview Reading:

Denham, J. (2018). Exercise and epigenetic inheritance of disease risk. *Acta Physiologica*. Blackwell Publishing Ltd.

Chapter 8: Special considerations

1. Solanki, G. (2012). International Journal of Pharmacological Research www. ssjournals. com. IJPR, 2(1), 63.

2. Jeffreys, R. M., Stepanchak, W., Lopez, B., Hardis, J., & Clapp III, J. F. (2006). Uterine blood flow during supine rest and exercise after 28 weeks of gestation. *BJOG: An International Journal of Obstetrics & Gynaecology*, 113(11), 1239-1247.

3. Colman-Brochu, S. (2004). Deep vein thrombosis in pregnancy. *MCN: The American Journal of Maternal/Child Nursing*, 29(3), 186-192.

4. Lee, N. M., & Saha, S. (2011). Nausea and vomiting of pregnancy. *Gastroenterology clinics of North America*, 40(2), 309–vii.

5. Dekkers, G. W. F., Broeren, M. A. C., Truijens, S. E. M., Kop, W. J., & Pop, V. J. M. (2020). Hormonal and psychological factors in nausea and vomiting during pregnancy. *Psychological Medicine*, 50(2), 229–236.

6. *Pavličev, M., Romero, R., & Mitteroecker, P. (2020). Evolution of the human pelvis and obstructed labor: new explanations of an old obstetrical dilemma. American journal of obstetrics and gynecology, 222(1), 3-16.*

7. Woodley, S. J., Lawrenson, P., Boyle, R., Cody, J. D., Mørkved, S., Kernohan, A., & Hay-Smith, E. J. C. (2020). Pelvic floor muscle training for preventing and treating urinary and faecal incontinence in antenatal and postnatal women. *Cochrane Database of Systematic Reviews*, (5).

8. Afshari, P., Dabagh, F., Iravani, M., & Abedi, P. (2017). Comparison of pelvic floor muscle strength in nulliparous women and those with normal vaginal delivery and cesarean section. *International Urogynecology Journal*, 28(8), 1171–1175.

9. Davenport, M. H., Marchand, A. A., Mottola, M. F., Poitras, V. J., Gray,

C. E., Garcia, A. J., ... & Skow, R. J. (2019). Exercise for the prevention and treatment of low back, pelvic girdle and lumbopelvic pain during pregnancy: a systematic review and meta-analysis. *British journal of sports medicine*, 53(2), 90-98

10. Owe, K. M., Bjelland, E. K., Stuge, B., Orsini, N., Eberhard-Gran, M., & Vangen, S. (2016). Exercise level before pregnancy and engaging in high-impact sports reduce the risk of pelvic girdle pain: a population-based cohort study of 39 184 women. *British journal of sports medicine*, 50(13), 817–822.

11. Liddle, S. D., & Pennick, V. (2015, September 30). Interventions for preventing and treating low-back and pelvic pain during pregnancy. *Cochrane Database of Systematic Reviews*. John Wiley and Sons Ltd.

12. Benjamin, D. R., van de Water, A. T. M., & Peiris, C. L. (2014). Effects of exercise on diastasis of the rectus abdominis muscle in the antenatal and postnatal periods: a systematic review. *Physiotherapy*, 100(1), 1–8.

13. Michalska, A., Rokita, W., Wolder, D., Pogorzelska, J., & Kaczmarczyk, K. (2018). Diastasis recti abdominis - A review of treatment methods. *Ginekologia Polska*. Via Medica.

14. Zheng, J., Wang, H., & Ren, M. (2017). Influence of exercise intervention on gestational diabetes mellitus: a systematic review and meta-analysis. *Journal of endocrinological investigation*, 40(10), 1027-1033.

15. Colberg, S. R. (2013). Prescribing physical activity to prevent and manage gestational diabetes. *World Journal of Diabetes*

16. Suzuki, S., Shinmura, H., & Kato, M. (2015). Maternal Uncontrolled Anxiety Disorders Are Associated With the Increased Risk of Hypertensive Disorders in Japanese Pregnant Women. *Journal of clinical medicine research*, 7(10), 791–794.

17. Barakat, R., Ruiz, J. R., & Lucia, A. (2009). Exercise during pregnancy and risk of maternal anaemia: a randomised controlled trial. *British journal of sports medicine*, 43(12), 954–956.

18. Price, B. B., Amini, S. B., & Kappeler, K. (2012). Exercise in pregnancy: Effect on fitness and obstetric outcomes - A randomized trial. *Medicine and Science in Sports and Exercise*.

19. Szymanski, L. M., & Satin, A. J. (2012). Strenuous exercise during pregnancy: is there a limit? *American Journal of Obstetrics and Gynecology*, 207(3), 179.e1-179.e6.

20. Kardel, K. R. (2005). Effects of intense training during and after pregnancy in top-level athletes. *Scandinavian Journal of Medicine and Science in Sports*, 15(2), 79–86.

Overview reading:

Woodley, S. J., Lawrenson, P., Boyle, R., Cody, J. D., Mørkved, S., Kernohan, A., & Hay-Smith, E. J. C. (2020). Pelvic floor muscle training for preventing and treating urinary and faecal incontinence in antenatal and postnatal women. Cochrane Database of Systematic Reviews.

Chapter 9: Postnatal life

1. Woodley, S. J., Boyle, R., Cody, J. D., Mørkved, S., & Hay-Smith, E. J. C. (2017). Pelvic floor muscle training for prevention and treatment of urinary and faecal incontinence in antenatal and postnatal women. *Cochrane Database of Systematic Reviews*, (12).

2. Van Geelen, H., Ostergard, D., & Sand, P. (2018). A review of the impact of pregnancy and childbirth on pelvic floor function as assessed by objective measurement techniques. *International Urogynecology Journal*, *29*(3), 327–338.

3. Bennett, R. J. (2014). Exercise for postnatal low back pain and pelvic pain. *Journal of the Association of Chartered Physiotherapists in Women's Health*, *115*, 14–21.

4. Cramp, A. G., & Bray, S. R. (n.d.). Understanding Exercise Self-Efficacy and Barriers to Leisure-Time Physical Activity Among Postnatal Women.

5. Davenport, M. H., McCurdy, A. P., Mottola, M. F., Skow, R. J., Meah, V. L., Poitras, V. J., … Ruchat, S. M. (2018). Impact of prenatal exercise on both prenatal and postnatal anxiety and depressive symptoms: A systematic review and meta-analysis. *British Journal of Sports Medicine*.

6. Saligheh, M., McNamara, B., & Rooney, R. (2016). Perceived barriers and enablers of physical activity in postpartum women: A qualitative approach. *BMC Pregnancy and Childbirth*.

7. Godin, G., Vezina, L., & Leclerc, O. (1974). *Factors Influencing Intentions of Pregnant Women to Exercise after Giving Birth. Source: Public Health Reports* (Vol. 104).

8. Demissie, Z. (2010). The Associations Between Physical Activity and Antepartum and Postpartum Depression. *UMI*.

9. Demissie, Z., Siega-Riz, A. M., Evenson, K. R., Herring, A. H., Dole, N., & Gaynes, B. N. (2013). Physical activity during pregnancy and postpartum depressive symptoms. *Midwifery*, *29*(2), 139–147.

10. Haruna, M., Watanabe, E., Matsuzaki, M., Ota, E., Shiraishi, M., Murayama, R., … Yeo, S. (2013). The effects of an exercise program on health-related quality of life in postpartum mothers: A randomized controlled trial. *Health*, *05*(03), 432–439.

11. Cramp, A. G., & Bray, S. R. (2010). Postnatal Women's Feeling State Responses to Exercise With and Without Baby. *Maternal and Child Health Journal*, *14*(3), 343–349.

12. Schmid, S., Stauffer, M., Jäger, J., List, R., & Lorenzetti, S. (2019). Sling-based infant carrying affects lumbar and thoracic spine neuromechanics during standing and walking. *Gait & Posture*, *67*, 172–180.

13. Lee, H., & Hong, K. H. (2017). Alteration of the Spine Shape Depending on the Wearing Method and Type of Baby Carrier. *Korean Journal of Human Ecology*, *26*(5), 435–444.

14. Chao Y. W., Hsiao R. H, Mao J W (2014), 'The Ergonomic Evaluations of Three Front Baby Carriers', Advances in Human Factors and Ergonomics

2014. Proceeding of the 5th AHFE Conference. 19-23 July 2014: 119 – 205.

15. Siddicky, S. F., Bumpass, D. B., Krishnan, A., Tackett, S. A., McCarthy, R. E., & Mannen, E. M. (2020). Positioning and baby devices impact infant spinal muscle activity. *Journal of Biomechanics*, *104*, 109741.

16. Galbally, M., van Rossum, E. F. C., Watson, S. J., de Kloet, E. R., & Lewis, A. J. (2019). Trans-generational stress regulation: Mother-infant cortisol and maternal mental health across the perinatal period. *Psychoneuroendocrinology*, *109*, 104374.

17. Afshari, P., Dabagh, F., Iravani, M., & Abedi, P. (2017). Comparison of pelvic floor muscle strength in nulliparous women and those with normal vaginal delivery and cesarean section. *International Urogynecology Journal*, *28*(8), 1171–1175.

18. Ghanbari Andarieh, M., Rani, V. M., & Hoseinpoor Heidary, F. (2016). Effectiveness of planned teaching programme on practice of post natal exercises among mothers who have undergone lower segment cesarean section. *Int J Reprod Contracept Obstet Gynecol*, *5*(11), 3782–3788

19. Benjamin, D. R., van de Water, A. T. M., & Peiris, C. L. (2014). Effects of exercise on diastasis of the rectus abdominis muscle in the antenatal and postnatal periods: a systematic review. *Physiotherapy*, *100*(1), 1–8.

20. Lim, S., Hill, B., Teede, H. J., Moran, L. J., & O'Reilly, S. (2020). An evaluation of the impact of lifestyle interventions on body weight in postpartum women: A systematic review and meta-analysis. *Obesity Reviews*, *21*(4).

21. Lovelady, C. (2011). Balancing exercise and food intake with lactation to promote post-partum weight loss. *Proceedings of the Nutrition Society*, *70*(2), 181–184.

22. Ferrari, N., Bae-Gartz, I., Bauer, C., Janoschek, R., Koxholt, I., Mahabir, E., … Graf, C. (2018). Exercise during pregnancy and its impact on mothers and offspring in humans and mice. *Journal of Developmental Origins of Health and Disease*, *9*(1), 63–76.

23. Reddish P, Fischer R, Bulbulia J. Let's Dance Together: Synchrony, Shared Intentionality and Cooperation. PLoS One [Internet]. 2013 Aug 7;8(8):e71182.

24. Dietz, P., Watson, E. D., Sattler, M. C., Ruf, W., Titze, S., & van Poppel, M. (2016). The influence of physical activity during pregnancy on maternal, fetal or infant heart rate variability: a systematic review. *BMC Pregnancy and Childbirth*, *16*(1), 326.

Overview Reading:

Ross, K. M., Carroll, J., Horvath, S., Hobel, C. J., Coussons-Read, M. E., & Dunkel Schetter, C. (2020). Immune epigenetic age in pregnancy and 1 year after birth: Associations with weight change. American Journal of Reproductive Immunology, 83(5), e13229.

Chapter 10: The next generation

1. McKenna, J. J., & Mosko, S. S. (1994). Sleep and arousal, synchrony and independence, among mothers and infants sleeping apart and together (same bed): an experiment in evolutionary medicine. *Acta Paediatrica*, *83*, 94-102.

2. Tonna, M., Marchesi, C., & Parmigiani, S. (2019). The biological origins of rituals: An interdisciplinary perspective. *Neuroscience & Biobehavioral Reviews*, *98*, 95–106.

3. Bergmeier, H., Paxton, S. J., Milgrom, J., Anderson, S. E., Baur, L., Hill, B., … Skouteris, H. (2020). Early mother-child dyadic pathways to childhood obesity risk: A conceptual model. *Appetite*, *144*, 104459

4. Bergmeier, H., Hill, B., Haycraft, E., Blewitt, C., Lim, S., Meyer, C., & Skouteris, H. (2020). Maternal body dissatisfaction in pregnancy, postpartum and early parenting: An overlooked factor implicated in maternal and childhood obesity risk. *Appetite*, *147*, 104525.

5. Afonso, L., Lopes, C., Severo, M., Santos, S., Real, H., Durão, C., … Oliveira, A. (2016). Bidirectional association between parental child-feeding practices and body mass index at 4 and 7 y of age. *The American Journal of Clinical Nutrition*, *103*(3), 861–867.

6. Evans, J., & Davies, B. (2010). Family, class and embodiment: why school physical education makes so little difference to post-school participation patterns in physical activity. *International Journal of Qualitative Studies in Education*, *23*(7), 765–784.

7. McLoone, P., & Morrison, D. S. (2014). Risk of child obesity from parental obesity: analysis of repeat national cross-sectional surveys. *The European Journal of Public Health*, *24*(2), 186–190.

8. Haire-Joshu, D., & Tabak, R. (2016). Preventing Obesity Across Generations: Evidence for Early Life Intervention. *Annual Review of Public Health*, *37*(1), 253–271.

9. Labayen, I., Medrano, M., Arenaza, L., Maíz, E., Osés, M., Martínez-Vizcaíno, V., … Ortega, F. B. (2020). Effects of Exercise in Addition to a Family-Based Lifestyle Intervention Program on Hepatic Fat in Children With Overweight. *Diabetes Care*, *43*(2), 306–313.

10. Lin, H., Hung, Y., Weng, S., Lee, P., & Sun, W. (2020). Effects of parent-based social media and moderate exercise on the adherence and pulmonary functions among asthmatic children. *The Kaohsiung Journal of Medical Sciences*, *36*(1), 62–70.

Overview reading:

Kincaid, H. J., Nagpal, R., & Yadav, H. (2020). Microbiome-immune-metabolic axis in the epidemic of childhood obesity: Evidence and opportunities. *Obesity Reviews*, *21*(2).

Chapter 11: Agents of change

1. McKenna, J., Naylor, P. J., & McDowell, N. (1998). Barriers to physical activity promotion by general practitioners and practice nurses. *British journal of sports medicine*, 32(3), 242-247.

2. Chatterjee, R., Chapman, T., Brannan, M. G., & Varney, J. (2017). GPs' knowledge, use, and confidence in national physical activity and health guidelines and tools: a questionnaire-based survey of general practice in England. *British Journal of General Practice*, 67(663), e668–e675.

3. England, N. H. S. (2016). Better births: Improving outcomes of maternity services in England-A five year forward view for maternity care. *London: NHS England*.

4. De Vivo, M., & Mills, H. (2019). "They turn to you first for everything": insights into midwives' perspectives of providing physical activity advice and guidance to pregnant women. *BMC pregnancy and childbirth*, 19(1), 462.

5. Dinwoodie, K., Moran, V. H., & Bramwell, R. (2001). Should midwives be teaching aquanatal exercise? *British Journal of Midwifery*, 9(5), 275–280.

6. World Health Organization. (2014). Toolkit for delivering the 5A's and 5R's brief tobacco interventions to TB patients in primary care.

Overview reading:

Yeates, T., Kolker, S., & Rezmovitz, J. (2020). I've stopped telling my patients to exercise. *Canadian Family Physician*.

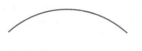

Index

Available from Pinter & Martin
*in the **Why it Matters** series*

Series editor: Susan Last

pinterandmartin.com